UNTOLD STORIES FROM THE IRON LUNG

Courageous True Tales of Six Polio Survivors Who Defied the Odds

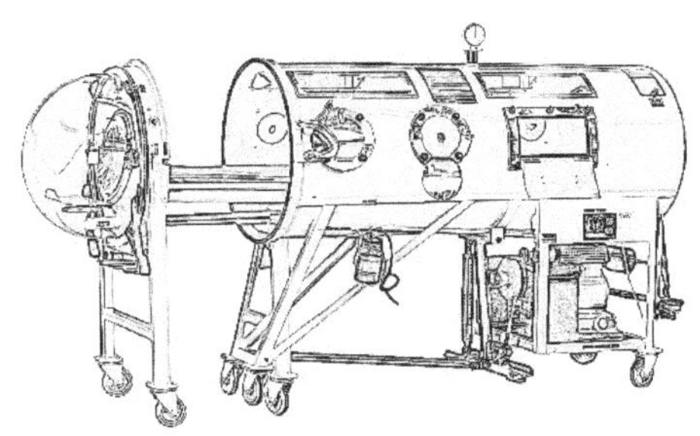

Ethan Hoover

Contents

Introduction

In medical history, few innovations have captured the essence of human resilience and ingenuity quite like the iron lung. The iron lung stands as a symbol of hope, survival, and the relentless pursuit of life against all odds.

Imagine a time when the danger of polio was endemic, casting a shadow of terror and uncertainty over communities around the world. In the early to mid-20th century, polio epidemics swept across continents, leaving a trail of devastation in their wake. Amidst the chaos and despair, a remarkable invention emerged; a contraption of steel and machinery that would come to define an era and transform the lives of those afflicted by the cruel hand of fate.

The iron lung, with its imposing presence and life-sustaining capabilities, became a beacon of hope for thousands grappling with the debilitating effects of respiratory paralysis. Developed in the 1920s by a team of pioneering minds at Harvard University, the iron lung represented a revolutionary leap forward in the treatment of respiratory conditions, particularly those caused by the poliovirus.

As the pages of history turned, the iron lung evolved from a crude apparatus into a marvel of modern engineering, embodying the relentless pursuit of innovation and the boundless potential of human creativity. From its humble beginnings as a makeshift plywood prototype to its mass production and distribution in the late 1930s, the iron lung emerged as a symbol of defiance in the face of adversity—a lifeline for those teetering on the brink of life and death.

Behind the cold steel and mechanical whirring lay stories of courage, resilience, and the triumph of the human spirit. Six individuals, bound together by the shared experience of survival, each bore witness to the transformative power of the iron lung in their lives. From the bustling streets of New York City to the cultural hub of Dallas Texas, their journeys stand as proofs of the agility of the human spirit and the enduring power of hope in trying times.

Paul Alexander, a polio survivor since 1952, found solace and sanctuary within the confines of his iron lung. Despite the passage of time, the unwavering spirit and determination of Alexander and five other individuals featured in this book serve as a reminder of the indomitable human will to persevere against all odds. As the pages of history turned, the iron lung evolved from a symbol of despair into a beacon of hope. In the following chapters, we will explore the untold stories of survival, resilience, and triumph that have shaped the legacy of the iron lung. From the laboratories of Harvard University to the bustling streets of New York City, the journey of the iron lung is a testament to the enduring power of human ingenuity and the indomitable spirit of the human heart.

The Iron Lung

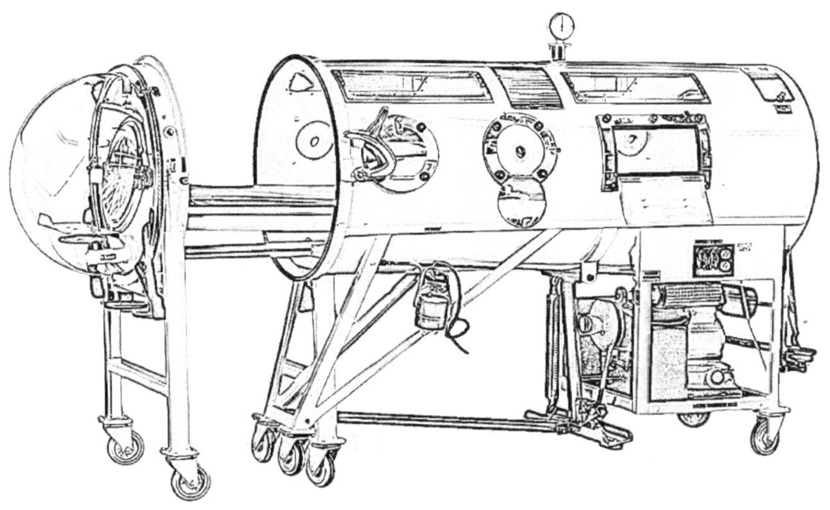

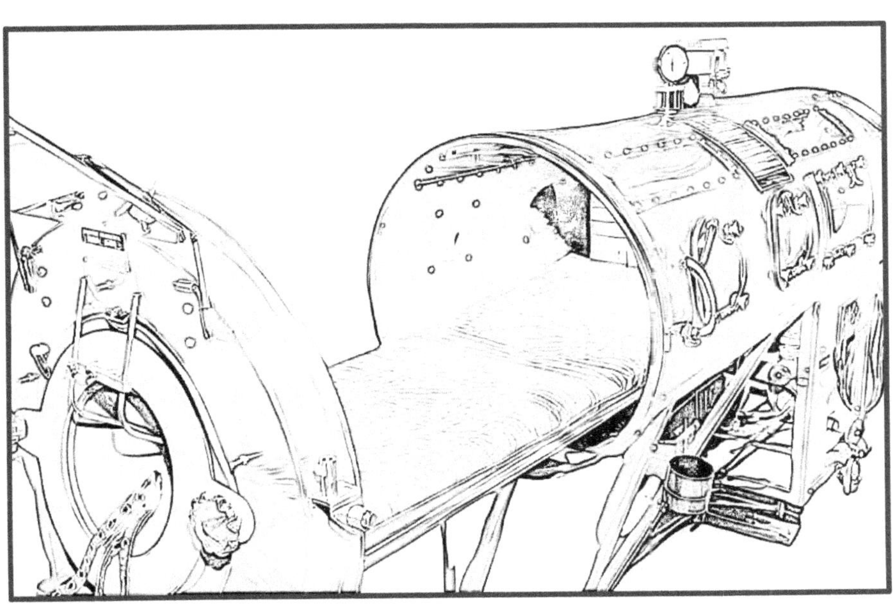

Part 1

Understanding the Machine and its Marvels

Chapter 1

What is an Iron Lung and How Does it Work?

Born out of necessity and ingenuity, this mechanical marvel stands as proof of humanity's resilience and innovation in the face of adversity. The concept of external negative pressure ventilation, the fundamental principle behind the iron lung, traces its roots back centuries. In 1670, John Mayow introduced the notion of negative pressure breathing, setting the stage for future breakthroughs in respiratory support. However, it wasn't until the early 20th century that this concept materialized into a tangible form of medical intervention.

In 1928, Philip Drinker and Louis Shaw unveiled the world's first practical iron lung at Boston Children's Hospital. Initially developed for the treatment of coal gas poisoning, the iron lung quickly gained renown as a lifesaving apparatus for individuals stricken with respiratory failure, particularly those afflicted by the devastating effects of poliomyelitis.

Design and Function

At its core, the iron lung is a marvel of engineering ingenuity. Consisting of a large horizontal cylinder, the apparatus envelops the patient's body while leaving the head exposed to the ambient air. The cylindrical chamber, typically made of steel rather than iron, is sealed to create an airtight environment conducive to respiratory manipulation.

The mechanics of the iron lung operate on the principle of external negative pressure ventilation (ENPV). Through a carefully orchestrated process, air pressure within the cylinder is meticulously regulated to induce inhalation and exhalation. As air is pumped out of the chamber, a slight vacuum is created, prompting the expansion of the patient's chest and facilitating the intake of oxygen-rich air. Conversely, when air is reintroduced into the chamber, the patient exhales, expelling carbon dioxide and waste gases from the lungs.

Evolution and Variations

In the years following its inception, the iron lung underwent significant refinement and innovation. John Haven Emerson introduced an enhanced version of the device in 1931, paving the way for wider accessibility and adoption. Concurrently, the *Both* respirator emerged as a cost-effective alternative to the Drinker model, offering a lighter and more portable solution for patients in need of respiratory support.

Moreover, advancements in miniaturization led to the development of smaller iterations of the iron lung, such as the Cuirass ventilator and Jacket ventilator. These compact variants, while retaining the essential principles of negative pressure ventilation, offered greater flexibility and comfort for patients undergoing treatment.

Method and Use

The utilization of the iron lung represents a convergence of medical science and compassionate care. For individuals afflicted with conditions ranging from polio to botulism, the device served as a beacon of hope in the heart of adversity. As patients were ensconced within the confines of the cylindrical chamber, a symphony of pneumatic motions controlled their respiratory rhythms, sustaining life where once there was peril.

Within the gloomy halls of polio wards during the mid-20th century, iron lungs stood as silent sentinels against the ravages of disease. As polio outbreaks swept across continents, these mechanical behemoths bore witness to both triumph and tragedy, offering solace to those ensnared in the grip of paralysis.

Legacy and Modern Applications

While the era of widespread iron lung usage has largely faded into memory, its legacy endures as evidence of mankind's resourcefulness and grit. In an age marked by technological marvels and medical breakthroughs, the iron lung stands as a poignant reminder of a bygone era.

Though relegated to the archives of medical history, the iron lung's impact reverberates through the corridors of time. In moments of crisis, such as the COVID-19 pandemic, echoes of its legacy resound, prompting reflection on the enduring power of innovation. As we look to the future, let us not forget the lessons imparted by the iron lung. In its embrace, we find not only the triumph of science but also the triumph of humanity against a deadly virus.

Chapter 2

Pioneers and Innovators of the Iron Lung

Few inventions in history have captured the imagination and revolutionized patient care quite like the iron lung. Born out of necessity and fueled by the relentless march of disease, the iron lung stands as a reminder of humanity's unwavering resolve to curb adversity. From its humble origins to its widespread adoption across the globe, the story of the iron lung is one of triumph over tragedy and hope over despair.

The Genesis of an Idea: From Antiquity to Modernity

The roots of the iron lung can be traced back through the accounts of the past, its origins intertwined with the timeless quest for developing viable solutions to combat respiratory disease. In 1670, English scientist John Mayow laid the groundwork for external negative pressure ventilation, envisioning a device that could pull air in and expel it from the lungs. Over the centuries, pioneers and visionaries alike toiled tirelessly to bring Mayow's vision to life, each contributing a piece to the puzzle of respiratory therapy.

In 1832, British physician John Dalziel unveiled the first negative pressure ventilator, setting the stage for a new era of medical innovation. Yet, it wasn't until the 20th century that the iron lung would emerge from the crucible of scientific inquiry, forever altering the landscape of respiratory care.

A Breath of Hope: The Drinker and Shaw Era

In the research laboratories of the Harvard School of Public Health, two visionary minds embarked on a journey that would change the course of medical history. In 1928, Philip Drinker and Louis Agassiz Shaw Jr., professors of industrial hygiene, unveiled the world's first iron lung.

Powered by an electric motor and equipped with air pumps scavenged from vacuum cleaners, the Drinker respirator breathed life into the lungs of its first patient—an eight-year-old girl on the brink of death from polio-induced respiratory paralysis. Her miraculous recovery sent shockwaves through the medical community, propelling the iron lung into the spotlight and igniting a wave of innovation and progress in its wake.

The Evolution of Innovation: From Drinker to Emerson

As the demand for respiratory therapy soared, so too did the need for innovation and progress in the realm of medical technology. In 1931, John Haven Emerson unveiled an improved and less expensive version of the iron lung, featuring a sliding bed and portal windows for enhanced patient care. Yet, Emerson's triumph was not without controversy, as legal battles over patent rights threatened to derail the march of progress.

In a landmark case that would shape the course of medical history, Emerson stood firm in his belief that life-saving technology should be freely available to all. His court victory paved the way for a new era of accessibility and affordability in respiratory care, ensuring that the benefits of the iron lung would reach those in need, regardless of their means.

A Global Phenomenon: The Both Respirator

As the specter of polio loomed large over communities around the world, the need for affordable and accessible respiratory therapy became more pressing than ever. In 1937, amidst an epidemic sweeping across Australia, biomedical engineer Edward Both answered the call, crafting a plywood marvel that would forever change the course of respiratory care.

The Both respirator, with its lightweight design and ease of construction, offered a lifeline to patients and practitioners alike, providing hope where once there was anguish. Lord Nuffield, moved by the plight of those suffering from respiratory paralysis, financed the production of thousands of Both respirators, ensuring that no corner of the globe would be untouched by the promise of breath.

The Legacy of Innovation: Looking to the Future

As we stand on the threshold of a new era in medical innovation, the legacy of the iron lung serves as a guiding light. From the bustling streets of Boston to the tranquil shores of Australia, the iron lung has left a mark on the pages of history, forever changing the way we think about respiratory care.

As we look to the future, let us draw inspiration from the pioneers and visionaries who came before us, forging a path forward guided by the principles of compassion, innovation, and solidarity. For in the face of adversity, we find our greatest strength, and in the pursuit of knowledge, we discover the power to change the world. The story of the iron lung is far from over—it is merely the beginning of a new chapter in the ongoing saga of human ingenuity and the relentless quest for advancement.

Part 2

**The Ravaging Polio
Epidemic and Advancement
of the Iron Lung**

Chapter 3

History of Polio

Polio, formally known as poliomyelitis, has left its mark on human history for millennia. Ancient Egyptian artifacts portray individuals with withered limbs and children reliant on canes, suggesting the presence of the disease in early civilizations. Even Emperor Claudius of Rome was believed to have been affected by polio during his childhood, leaving him with a lifelong limp. However, the disease remained largely undocumented until the 18th century when Sir Walter Scott's detailed account hinted at a retrospective diagnosis of polio.

Throughout history, polio carried various names reflecting its devastating impact: Dental Paralysis, Infantile Spinal Paralysis, and Regressive Paralysis, among others. Despite these observations, it wasn't until the 19th century that physicians began clinically documenting cases, with Jakob Heine providing the first medical report in 1840.

Emergence of Epidemics

Major polio outbreaks were virtually unheard of before the 20th century. However, by the early 1900s, localized epidemics began surfacing in Europe and the United States. The disease's swift transmission and unpredictable onset struck fear into communities, leading to widespread panic and drastic measures to contain its spread.

The infamous 1916 polio epidemic in New York marked a turning point in public awareness. With over 27,000 cases and 7,130 deaths in the United

States alone, the epidemic triggered mass hysteria, prompting cities to implement quarantines and citizens to flee to rural areas. The relentless summer outbreaks persisted, peaking in the 1940s and 1950s, culminating in the devastating 1949 epidemic with over 42,000 reported cases and thousands of deaths.

The Polio Plague: Fear and Hesitation

The polio virus struck indiscriminately, afflicting individuals regardless of age or socioeconomic status. Its rapid onset and varying severity left communities reeling in uncertainty. The fear of contracting polio was engraved in people's hearts, compelling families to adopt ineffective preventive measures and shun public gatherings.

The seasonal nature of polio outbreaks, primarily in late spring and summer, fueled misconceptions about its transmission, with flies and mosquitoes often blamed. Despite efforts to curb the disease, including the widespread use of the pesticide DDT, the number of cases continued to escalate, reaching a peak of 52,000 in 1952.

Innovations in Treatment and Prevention

The medical community grappled with the lack of effective treatments for polio during the early 20th century. Bizarre remedies, including oxygen therapy and poultices, offered little relief to patients. However, pioneering efforts led to significant breakthroughs in polio management.

The introduction of the iron lung in 1928 revolutionized respiratory care for paralyzed patients, offering a glimmer of hope amidst the epidemic. Despite its size and cost, the iron lung saved countless lives, albeit with limitations. Alongside respiratory aids, such as the Bragg-Paul Pulsator, researchers explored passive immunotherapy and surgical interventions to mitigate the disease's debilitating effects.

The Kenny Regimen

Sister Elizabeth Kenny's groundbreaking approach to polio treatment challenged conventional wisdom, advocating for early mobilization and physical therapy instead of immobilization. Her innovative methods, emphasizing hot packs and exercise, transformed the landscape of polio rehabilitation, paving the way for modern rehabilitation therapy.

The Path to Vaccination

Amidst the despair of relentless polio outbreaks, the quest for a vaccine emerged as a glimmer of hope. The tireless efforts of researchers, including John Enders and Jonas Salk, culminated in the development of the injectable polio vaccine in 1955. Albert Sabin's oral vaccine followed suit, offering a comprehensive solution to polio prevention.

The rigorous testing and validation process underscored the monumental achievement of vaccine development, heralding the beginning of the end of polio's reign of terror. Despite lingering challenges, including vaccine distribution and public acceptance, the successful eradication of polio in most parts of the world stands as a victory for all.

The history of polio epitomizes humanity's resilience in the face of adversity. From ancient civilizations to modern societies, the specter of polio has spurred innovation, solidarity, and compassion. While the scars of polio outbreaks endure in the collective memory, they also serve as a reminder of the indomitable spirit that unites us in the pursuit of a healthier, more equitable world.

As we confront new challenges in the form of emerging diseases, the lessons of polio remain etched in our collective consciousness, offering hope and inspiration in the quest for a brighter tomorrow. In the words of P.D. Howe, "Hope grows that the end of this epidemic may be in sight... But these things only mean that we are entering a new phase," reaffirming our commitment to overcoming adversity and embracing the promise of a healthier future.

Chapter 4

The Psychological and Social Impact of Polio

Polio, once a dreaded scourge of humanity, not only exacted a toll on the physical health of its victims but also left profound psychological and social scars in its wake. In this chapter, we delve into the multifaceted impact of polio on individuals, families, and societies during the era when the disease reigned unchecked.

The Invisible Terror: Psychological Trauma of Polio

Polio's insidious nature, characterized by its sudden onset and unpredictable outcomes, instilled a deep sense of fear and anxiety in those vulnerable to its grasp. The specter of paralysis loomed large, casting a shadow of uncertainty over individuals and communities alike. For parents, the fear of their child falling victim to the disease was a constant source of anguish, permeating every aspect of daily life.

The psychological trauma inflicted by polio extended far beyond the physical manifestations of the disease. The threat of permanent disability, coupled with the lack of effective treatments, fueled a sense of helplessness and despair among patients and their loved ones. The sudden loss of mobility and independence shattered dreams and aspirations, leaving individuals grappling with a profound sense of loss and grief.

Moreover, the stigma associated with polio compounded the psychological burden borne by its victims. Society's perception of disability as a mark of weakness or inferiority presides over those afflicted by the disease, exacerbating feelings of isolation and marginalization. The pervasive fear of contagion further fueled social ostracization, leading to the alienation of polio survivors from their communities.

The Burden of Care: Impact on Families and Caregivers

Polio's toll extended beyond the individual affected to encompass the entire family unit. The relentless demands of caregiving placed immense strain on families already grappling with the emotional and financial burdens of the disease. Parents watched helplessly as their children battled the ravages of polio, navigating a landscape fraught with uncertainty and despair.

The practical challenges of caring for a polio survivor were manifold, requiring round-the-clock attention and support. From assisting with daily activities to navigating the complexities of medical treatment, caregivers bore the weight of responsibility with unwavering dedication and resilience. Yet, amidst the demands of caregiving, families grappled with feelings of guilt, frustration, and exhaustion, struggling to reconcile their own needs with those of their loved ones.

Furthermore, the financial implications of polio placed significant strain on families already teetering on the brink of poverty. The exorbitant costs of medical care, coupled with the loss of income due to disability, pushed many families to the brim of destitution, perpetuating a cycle of economic hardship and social inequality.

A World Transformed: Social Implications of Polio

The pervasive impact of polio reverberated throughout society, reshaping social norms, attitudes, and perceptions in profound ways. The emergence of polio epidemics spurred unprecedented levels of public mobilization and awareness, galvanizing communities to confront the looming threat of the disease head-on. Yet, amidst the collective response to polio, deep-seated prejudices and misconceptions persisted, perpetuating a cycle of fear and discrimination.

Polio's legacy extended beyond the confines of the individual. The prevalence of disability challenged prevailing notions of normalcy and conformity, forcing society to confront its own biases and preconceptions. Yet, despite efforts to promote inclusivity and acceptance, the specter of polio widely wrecked the lives of those it affected, relegating them to the margins of society.

Moreover, the social stigma associated with polio perpetuated a culture of silence and shame, inhibiting open dialogue and discourse surrounding the disease. Polio survivors grappled with feelings of isolation and alienation in navigating a world laden with barriers and obstacles. The absence of societal support and understanding further compounded the challenges faced by individuals living with the long-term effects of polio, perpetuating a cycle of invisibility and neglect.

Coping Mechanisms and Resilience: Finding Hope in Adversity

Amidst the darkness of despair, polio survivors and their families demonstrated remarkable resilience and fortitude in the face of adversity. From forging networks of support to advocating for greater awareness and inclusivity, individuals affected by polio refused to be defined by their circumstances, embracing hope and possibility amid hardship.

Coping mechanisms varied widely among polio survivors, ranging from peer support groups to creative outlets such as art and music therapy. The power of community proved instrumental in fostering a sense of belonging and solidarity, offering a lifeline of support in times of need. Through shared experiences and mutual understanding, polio survivors found solace and strength in the bonds forged amidst adversity.

Moreover, the advent of rehabilitation therapy and assistive technologies heralded a new era of empowerment and independence for individuals living with the long-term effects of polio. From adaptive mobility devices to innovative rehabilitation techniques, advancements in medical science offered new avenues for reclaiming autonomy and dignity in the face of disability.

The echoes of polio's grip on the past resonate deeply, a poignant reminder of the tenacity of the human spirit in the face of hardship. Where despair might have taken root, tales of courage, compassion, and solidarity bloomed, defying anguish with the transformative power of hope.

As we reflect on the legacy of polio, we are reminded of the enduring importance of empathy, understanding, and inclusivity in our collective journey toward healing and reconciliation. The lessons learned from the psychological and social impact of polio offer valuable insights into the complexities of human experience, inspiring us to embrace diversity, celebrate resilience, and forge a more compassionate and inclusive world for all.

Chapter 5

Evolution of the Iron Lung

As polio epidemics swept across the globe, the iron lung, a revolutionary invention born in the 1920s at Harvard University by Philip Drinker, Louis Agassiz Shaw, and James Wilson, offered a beacon of hope to those stricken by the disease's devastating effects, particularly respiratory paralysis.

The early iron lungs, characterized by their cumbersome design and mechanical complexity, represented a groundbreaking advancement in medical technology. Powered by electric motors and vacuum cleaners, these negative pressure ventilators mimicked the physiological process of breathing, enabling patients to draw air into their lungs and expel carbon dioxide.

Challenges and Innovations

Despite its life-saving potential, the early iron lungs posed significant challenges in terms of accessibility, affordability, and portability. The sheer size and weight of the machines rendered them impractical for widespread use, particularly in resource-limited settings and regions affected by polio outbreaks.

However, the relentless pursuit of innovation and adaptation led to significant advancements in the design and functionality of the iron lung. Engineers and inventors sought to streamline the manufacturing process, reduce costs, and enhance patient accessibility, driving the evolution of the iron lung into a more efficient and user-friendly device.

One notable example of innovation came from Edward Both, an engineer who developed a prototype iron lung using plywood during a polio outbreak in Australia. This makeshift device demonstrated the potential for rapid deployment and construction, paving the way for future iterations of the iron lung that prioritized accessibility and efficiency.

Mass Distribution and Utilization

The late 1930s marked a turning point in the mass distribution and utilization of iron lungs, with as many as 1,200 individuals in the United States alone relying on these life-saving devices for respiratory support. The widespread availability of iron lungs offered a glimmer of hope for polio survivors grappling with the debilitating effects of respiratory paralysis.

However, not every polio sufferer was fortunate enough to regain breathing function within a few weeks. For some individuals, permanent muscle and lung damage necessitated long-term or permanent reliance on iron lungs for respiratory support. Despite the challenges and limitations associated with their use, iron lungs represented a lifeline for those in need of respiratory assistance.

The Era of Obsolescence

The advent of the polio vaccine and advancements in mechanical ventilation heralded the gradual obsolescence of the iron lung in the latter half of the 20th century. As polio cases dwindled and modern ventilators emerged as more efficient and versatile alternatives, the once indispensable iron lung faded into obscurity.

Yet, for a few polio survivors like Paul Alexander, the iron lung remained a vital lifeline, symbolizing resilience and defiance in the face of adversity. Despite the challenges of maintaining and repairing these aging devices, individuals like Alexander continued to rely on their iron lungs for respiratory support, steadfast in their belief in the therapeutic benefits of these historic machines.

The Legacy of Innovation

While modern ventilators have supplanted iron lungs as the primary means of respiratory support in intensive care units and emergency wards, the spirit of innovation and resilience embodied by the iron lung endures.

The iron lung's remarkable evolution encapsulates the transformative power of medical innovation on human health. Birthed from a humble plywood prototype, it transcended its makeshift origins to become a symbol of hope and survival in the face of polio's devastation. This human ingenuity stands as a stark reminder that even the most daunting challenges can be met with solutions born from relentless pursuit and unwavering optimism.

Looking to the Future

As we reflect on the evolution of the iron lung, we are reminded of the enduring importance of innovation, collaboration, and compassion in the pursuit of medical progress. While the era of the iron lung may have drawn to a close, its legacy continues to inspire future generations of researchers, inventors, and healthcare professionals to push the boundaries of possibility and redefine the landscape of medical care.

As we stand on the threshold of a new era of medical innovation, guided by the lessons of the past and fueled by the promise of the future, we honor the legacy of the iron lung and celebrate the spirit of resilience and hope that it represents. In the journey ahead, may we continue to embrace the challenges of the unknown with courage, determination, and unwavering resolve, knowing that the pursuit of knowledge and healing is a timeless endeavor that knows no bounds.

Part 3

Survival Story of Six Famous Polio Victims

Chapter 6

Adolf Ratzka's Story

"The worth of a life should not be determined by what we can 'achieve' in the eyes of society but by the satisfaction we find in pursuing chosen goals and realizing dreams limited only by the risks that others may impose on us against our will." — Adolf Ratzka

Against the flickering glow of black-and-white images depicting rows of coffin-like iron cylinders, a pajama-clad little figure gazes through an expressionless face yet eyes hinting at bewilderment. At age 5 in 1948, a fire ravaged Adolf's Hamburg neighborhood; he and his neighbors took temporary refuge in hospital wards filled with breathing machines. Though not yet

stricken himself, early childhood memories lingered
of machines automatically pumping air into withered
lungs. A decade hence, post-war life in shattered
Germany held greater horrors in store for him than
his war times experiences.

Adolf dared an impulsive jump into lake waters
during a 1958 family vacation in Sweden—the last
time his athletic teenager legs would spring freely.
Bobbing back to the surface, he felt strangely
hampered trying to paddle ashore. Doctors assessed
his sudden paralysis as beyond their capacity to
ameliorate. With polio rapidly paralyzing chest
muscles, only immediate enclosure inside an iron lung
offered any probability of sustaining fragile life
functions.

Transported over 250 miles to the University Hospital
in Lund, Adolf's parents kept an anxious bedside vigil.
Trapped motionless on his back, the athletic kid

acutely sensed each breath becoming shallower, increasingly starved of oxygen. Attendants hurriedly prepared the respiration chamber for the now critically-struggling patient. His mother gently squeezed her son's hand in desperate reassurance before assistants encased his body, aside from the head, inside the confining steel column. Faint memories of laughing children peering from similar metallic cylinders now felt devastatingly ominous rather than merely puzzling. This was surely no laughing matter.

Nine feet of bolted steel plates sealed Adolf into isolation without the capacity to see family keeping hopeful watch. As the motorized pumps began cycling, he anxiously wondered if the experiment might yet succeed despite long odds. Had he infected his lungs fatally beyond recovery? Might today instead mark the commencement of life bound permanently to an apparatus embodying captivity itself? Either prospect loomed devastating. Yet suspense concluded as air gently filled his chest despite paralysis—breath restored by mechanical means with his parents just out of sight. Ensconced securely inside, Adolf's gaze surveyed the exterior of his new metal abode while pondering unanswerable questions about an uncertain future now dependent upon this nineteenth-century invention.

Lasting Impacts: Defining Moments

Few life events parade consciousness more profoundly than staring mortality in the face while detained inside a metal wall tirelessly breathing for you. Only a few people would expect a peaceful summer adventure to brutally reshape their identity within minutes. Even six decades later, Adolf distinctly recalls the initial ten seconds of air starvation while his paralyzed lungs floundered while trying in vain to inflate. Though spared a suffocating death, the enveloping steel column would dominate nearly all facets of his existence during five prime years when his peers moved unencumbered into discovering life's new phases. Craving even modest mobility ultimately motivated him to learn how to breath independently using adapted body mechanics. But regaining his liberty came at the cost of formidable sacrifice.

Independence proved fleeting upon trading the iron lung's confines for the liberation of a wheelchair. Contracting bone tuberculosis resulting from lengthy immobility mandated two full body casts and another year immobilized—this time horizontal and cage-free yet still breath-short. Removed from casts, atrophied limbs could no longer propel a wheelchair or transfer to a bed. Few rehabilitation options existed for someone without the use of any extremity who nevertheless sought autonomy and typical student pursuits. Though foiled repeatedly in ambitions for independence and career, Adolf's irrepressible drive fueled ingenious alternative strategies and advocacy benefitting multitudes lacking his fortitude.

Journey Through Dark Places

During four arduous years spanning ages 17-21, hospital institutionalization reimposed cruel constraints on hard-won freedoms. Sharing quarters with elderly inhabitants abbreviated remaining vestiges of independence and dignity. Youthful mentality clashed against geriatric ward routines strictly regimenting tedious unchanging days.

Nursing staff dismissed requests for recreational diversion between mandatory times fixed for rising, meals, therapies, and sleep. Programmed days held scant stimulation save occasional family visits and glimpses of trees through windows taunting immobility. Reading or radio provided Adolf's only extracurricular fulfillment during the monotonous days blending one into the next. Four times weekly he endured painful stretching sessions trying to prevent his limbs from permanently freezing. Monotonous activities could not balance the despair at being stranded far from the world of the moving and breathing.

Liberation arrived unexpectedly upon a doctor inquiring if Adolf might welcome transferring somewhere enabling more youthful company and pursuits. Adolf leaped at the opportunity without hesitation. Thus, in the summer of 1966, he voyaged across continents to launch the next chapter of his remarkable life at sunny UCLA in California. Little did he know that not only the climate awaited drastic change. A fascinating journey into the disability rights revolution loomed just ahead for this venturesome young man positioned at the right time at the right frontier of history.

Finding Purpose on Campuses

Adolf's reputedly stubborn disposition surely assisted in pivoting his life's trajectory positively, despite having numerous physical setbacks. Even lengthy hospitalization could not quash his visions of university studies previously commenced in Sweden when healthier. Providentially the state of California sponsored a program enabling Adolf's enrollment at UCLA for regular coursework and campus residential living. This government-funded support furnished stipends for personal care assistants facilitating requisite daily aid including dressing, wheelchair maneuvering, and even notetaking for academic sessions.

For the first time since tragedy severed his boyhood, Adolf found himself immersed joyfully in college atmospheres bustling with kindreds his age. No locked wards or age gaps separated him from the climate of growth and discovery characterizing university environments. Back home in Sweden, only isolation and boredom awaited should his paralysis progress further. Changing location increased Adolf's chances to thrive without needing special assistance.

Typical student diversions like parties or clubs mattered less to Adolf than diligently reading through his course content. Psychology and economics classes illuminated society's inner workings, although adjustments were necessary for someone lacking limb function. Adolf appreciated UCLA's early efforts at accessibility accommodation decades before disability laws emerged. Still, struggling to manage heavy texts or scribble exam essays using an unwieldy mouth stick strained patience during long study hours.

Five years immersed in the University of California's cosmopolitan hodgepodge fortified Adolf's invaluable preparation for an upcoming pivotal role amid an about-to-ignite revolution. Fate situated him perfectly for engaging with the disability rights eruption about to remake campus life dramatically for generations to come.

Encountering the Independent Living Movement

When Adolf crossed paths with the pioneering Rolling Quads wheelchair brigade who commandeered societal change at UC Berkeley in the 1960s-70s, the philosophies they modeled altered his path permanently. Radical new concepts took shape before his eyes, initiated by those who refused to accept constraints on maximum participation and inclusion with non-disabled populations.

In May 1973, Adolf visited the Berkeley campus Harbor House residence where wheelchair-using students Ed Roberts and John Hessler pioneered revolutionizing approaches for managing quadriplegia independently while attending university. Staff provided personal care assistance while treating residents according to their preferences rather than institutional control. The novel philosophy emphasized wisdom over professional dominance across life decisions—an attitude shift rippling into the wider culture at large. This kernel of revelation during a single Harbor House encounter germinated Adolf's destiny henceforth as a trailblazer in spreading powerful sovereign values throughout multiple nations.

Just down the block, Rolling Quads colleagues began organizing a grassroots resource hub run by and for disabled students themselves rather than providers or doctors. The Center for Independent Living filled needs ranging from attendant referrals to exam accommodations or wheelchair repairs. By offering peer support, the group sought to shift negative cultural stereotyping of disability while maximizing autonomy. The pioneers clung to their hard-won campus freedoms while reaching to pull up oppressed comrades still trapped in the ugly status quo. Their example compelled Adolf to expand the vision.

Two pivotal ideas undergirded the independent living paradigm rapidly gaining authority as disenfranchised students claimed control. Firstly, people with similar disabilities provide the best counsel about life dilemmas—no one else comprehends internally as peers do. Secondly, insiders should rightfully determine their own lifestyle decisions rather than doctors or authorities. This transfer of self-direction from the medical system to the individual involved, utterly transformed Adolf's outlook and unleashed his advocacy gifts benefitting multitudes worldwide.

Charting an Advocacy Course

Adolf's eventual migration overseas prepared perfect conditions for transplanting Berkeley's theories to Sweden's barren disability rights. Fortuitously, California hosted the 1972 World Institute on Disability conference where Adolf gained insights about barrier removal from international perspectives. The summer 1973 Berkeley visit offered another revelation in possibilities. Lingering two months stateside after the pivotal introduction to Ed Roberts further expanded Adolf's awareness before returning home. He felt compelled towards activism to update his native country's archaic policies after exposure to groundbreaking alternatives.

Back in Europe, Adolf enrolled in a Swedish university's innovative educational program tailored to students with extensive disabilities. However, campus life still mandated residing in a locked nursing facility with elderly inhabitants, the daily undoing of personal independence so prized in California. Keen to import radical changes, Adolf soon rallied supporters towards building Sweden's initial Center for Independent Living, offering peer counseling and de-medicalized living options.

Adolf became further galvanized after an invitation to a 1977 disability activism summit in England. Though a painful bone disease increasingly hampered Adolf's torso movement, he nevertheless joined the notorious Wade House protest where attendees barricaded inside a residential institution to expose egregious human rights violations. Dramatic headlines delivered public outrage plus government scrutiny after shocking media footage revealed residents confined nude and neglected. Alongside counterparts like Ed Roberts or Judy Heumann, Adolf strategized how to transition institutionalized oppressions into progressive supports for self-driven community integration.

Swedish authorities cautiously took notice of Adolf's fiercely critical advocacy upon returning home, while counterparts privately admired his audacity in questioning the systemic status quo. In 1981 he co-founded STIL (the Stockholm Cooperative for Independent Living), the nation's first independent living cooperative, securing public funding for personal assistants and facilitating full social inclusion regardless of paralysis. STIL's groundbreaking success seeded parallel Swedish centers supporting customized living options as promotional efforts dispelled skepticism. Adolf's visibility as an independent quadriplegic citizen traversing Stockholm's urban landscape delivered a powerful message that disability need not equate to helplessness. However, the personal assistance model required relentless defense.

Over decades Adolf sharpened their rhetorical skills in defending disability rights locally and abroad whether addressing politicians, academics, or NGOs. His incisive intellect and trilingual eloquence commanded attention across mediums such as articles, speeches, interviews, or advisory councils. A prolific lecturer and networker, Adolf moved easily between grassroots activists and national platforms despite spinal fragility increasingly constricting his breathing. Traveling widely, he leveraged connections and insights to coax incremental disability justice gains throughout European bureaucracies mired in outdated custodial approaches.

Combating complacency with political savvy and legal pressures, Adolf continually educated stakeholders regarding policy gaps between paralysis rhetoric and daily civil rights realities. Whether lifting the visibility of disabled women's unmet needs, establishing Sweden's first personal assistance user cooperative, or co-founding an international disability human rights defenders' league, Adolf led courageously by example, never expecting others to take risks he would not try as well. After escaping two untimely brushes with

death in early years, Adolf dared a purposeful third
act defending liberties for multitudes lacking his
perseverance for emancipation.

An Unfinished Revolution

"Disability rights advocacy is like gardening," Adolf is
fond of reminding, "weeds always grow back requiring
continual diligence to not lose hard-won ground." As
movements evolve, Adolf believes unity is essential to
preserve founding values against institutionalization.
He contends that success embedded Independent
Living Councils into establishment bureaucracies,
eroding their bite by becoming too allied with funders.
Over time US disability nonprofits retreated from the
barricades into comfortable yet diluted roles
endorsing the status quo.

Having followed Sweden's independent living
trajectory since helping launch the maiden resource
center in 1979, Adolf charts similar patterns of radical

initiative surrendering progressive gains as the establishment embraces. Visionary firebrands tone down abrasiveness as erstwhile outlaws gain seats at bureaucratic tables. Adolf himself contributed through decades in committee posts consulting supportive political allies. Yet alongside high-level visibility, he still asserts that "rights on paper alone change nothing without enforcement." Fierce advocacy must press on.

Approaching age 80 and increasingly limited physically, Adolf continues advancing disability rights locally and abroad despite relying now on ventilators to aid waning pulmonary capacities. In terms of unrealized movement aims, he stresses the UN Convention on Disability Rights has achieved little since most nations ignore enforcement obligations. Similarly, Sweden failed to adopt requisite binding measures to implement paper guarantees. He believes pivoting from rhetorical rights language to practical governmental accountability remains imperative going forward. Litigation frequently proves the only equally powerful lever against bureaucratic inertia.

Today, from his home offices in Stockholm, Adolf collaborates with international colleagues through online networks like the European Network on Independent Living where he formerly served as chair and president. Always reaching out to empower upcoming activists, Adolf reminds it remains difficult growing up disabled in cultures devaluing lives deemed unproductive. Gathering young leaders prevents isolation while conveying "nothing about us without us" wisdom to counter internalized oppression. Despite frustration at plodding political progress, Adolf continues exerting a profound influence through his steely-eyed advocacy.

A Living Legacy

In 2048 the world will mark the 100th anniversary of the iron lung's miraculous respiratory redemption. By then Adolf will have breathed free of its confines for 90 years since the warm Swedish lake waters turned perilous in 1958. Few individuals owe their lives more literally to Philip Drinker and Louis Shaw's crude metallic contraption than the countless thousands rescued from paralytic oblivion during the 20th century's viral scourges.

Perhaps, Adolf Ratzka's most enduring legacies lies in refusing to relinquish independence even when breath itself grew scarce for quadriplegics before ventilators. Though initially restored by the iron lung's mechanical marvel, Adolf prized liberty too highly to remain hostage indefinitely. Through summoning extraordinary fortitude and creativity from broken places, his example shines as a triumph over recurring forces trying to bend lives towards insignificance.

Despite waging a lifetime's battle against recurring illness and constraint, Adolf lifted multitudes by championing disability pride and peer support. His living legacy continues advancing human rights for those relegated to margins by ableist indifference. Now 78 years along his unsought journey inside a body with an unclear prognosis, Adolf's breath may perhaps grow short again. Yet the formidable influence of his vision and voice shows no signs of abating.

All who care about inclusive communities enabling self-driven participation owe gratitude to this defiant pioneer for much of yesterday's impossible becoming today possible. By embodying the words inscribed upon Sweden's Parliament wall which first welcomed Adolf's wheelchair half a century ago, "Only a free and enlightened people preserve their liberty forever", he set captives free generation after generation. The breathtaking view from here remains steeped in Adolf Ratzka's stubborn nonconformity in lifting outliers.

Chapter 7

Mona Jean Randolph's Story

The screeching of metal echoed through the small wood-paneled bedroom as Mark Randolph wheeled an antique iron lung to the side of the bed. His wife Mona lay calmly beneath the white sheets, the rise and fall of her chest faint without the iron lung's assistance. Mark carefully opened the coffin-like machine, releasing trapped air with a hiss. Mona gave him a tired smile as he gently moved her legs, then torso inside. After 82 years together, guiding Mona into her metal cocoon had become routine, though no less harrowing. Once she was settled, he slowly closed the heavy lid until only her head peered out. Mona took a long, deep breath as the iron lung roared to life, the motorized pump creating negative pressure to expand her lungs. Though muffled within her metal shell, her voice rang clearly. "Goodnight my love, see you in the morning." Mark smiled, patting the machine affectionately. "Sleep well, darling. I'll be here when you wake."

As Mark climbed into bed, he marveled at his beloved wife sleeping peacefully in a relic from the 1940s polio epidemic. Mona was one of the last people on Earth who still relied on an iron lung. While most considered the archaic device an antique curiosity, for Mona it was life support; a yellow submarine granting her breath where her body failed. Mark often wondered at the twists and turns that brought them together. How did a prim Kansas farm girl wind up finding love in the arms of her iron lung? Now, as the shadows of mortality crept over them, he found himself contemplating the purpose behind Mona's remarkable life. There were so many questions he still longed to ask her. What gave her the perseverance to fight for breath and dignity for over 60 years? How did she maintain such vibrant faith while trapped in a metal coffin each night? In the morning light, he resolved to record Mona's incredible story before time robbed them of the chance. Her life was a testament to the resilience of the human spirit. She deserved for her story to be known.

The Early Years

Mona Jean Halliburton entered the world on August 26, 1936. The tiny, pink-faced infant with a shock of dark hair was born to Elmer and Mary Halliburton on their farm 10 miles outside of Paola, Kansas. She was the third of four daughters, surrounded by a menagerie of animals and wide-open pastures. Her father was a taciturn man who toiled from dawn to dusk tending crops and livestock. Though he loved his girls, he believed a woman's role was to marry young and maintain the home. Mary glided effortlessly between farm chores, whipping up hearty meals from garden-fresh produce and mending overalls worn thin from work. Though lacking formal education, she had sharp wits and a vibrant laugh that penetrated the quiet countryside.

As a young child, Mona trailed after her mother's skirt, mimicking her chores and mannerisms. She basked in Mary's affectionate praise at each new domestic skill mastered. But while she enjoyed cooking with her mother, Mona's heart pulled her toward the fields, where her father worked the land from the back of a plow horse. She envied her older sisters coming home sweat-stained and grass-stained from adventures in the woods and creeks crisscrossing their property. Though Elmer dismissed such unladylike amusements, Mary recognized her daughter's restless spirit. When chores allowed, she shooed the girl outdoors to run wild.

By age five, Mona could ride and care for horses, and milk cows, and identify all manner of crops and wildlife on the land she loved. Her curiosity and intelligence also shone through her schoolwork, where she devoured books on history, science, religion, and poetry. She wrote her first poem in second grade, describing the blazing colors of a summer sunset.

As she grew older, Mona's ill-fitting role as a farmer's daughter chafed. expected to stay inside practicing wifely duties while her heart longed for open skies and new horizons. The summer after eighth-grade graduation, she tearfully confessed her intentions to leave the family farm and continue school in the city. Elmer scowled in disapproval, lecturing her on the foolishness of girls seeking education and careers. But Mary read the conviction in her daughter's eyes. Taking her husband's rough hand, she reminded him that their Mona had gifts beyond their small community. With reluctant blessings, they sent their bright-eyed fourteen-year-old to live with her aunt and uncle in Kansas City to attend high school.

The City

For a farm girl raised in isolation, the sights and sounds of the big city were overwhelming. Electric lights, automobiles, and towering buildings dazzled her senses after years spent surrounded by cornfields. Mona attended classes at Northeast High School, struggling to concentrate with the rumble of trolleys and traffic outside. She dove into her books at night to understand this new urban landscape, reading about the Great Depression, World Wars, and advances in science and technology she had never known on the farm.

Outside school, Mona explored her new home with boundless energy. She and her cousin Martha spent long afternoons wandering the city on foot and streetcar. They window-shopped downtown stores, gazing at fine ladies in smart dresses and stylish hats so different from their homespun frocks. On weekends they packed sandwiches and took the long trolley ride to Swope Park. There they lazed in the sun, watching white sailboats skim across the lake. As her world expanded far beyond the confines she knew, so too did Mona's dreams for the future.

As high school graduation neared, Mona pictured herself as one of those sophisticated city women. Her teachers noted her talent for writing during a senior English project. Perhaps she could move to New York City and work for a lady's magazine! But practicality prevailed, and soon Mona found herself enrolled in a business college to train as a secretary. She rationalized that an office job allowed time to nurture artistic pursuits while providing a steady income.

In the fall of 1955, Mona started work at United Missouri Bank. She quickly mastered shorthand and typing skills in the steno pool. But her sharp business acumen shone, and soon she took over payroll operations. She delighted in dressing smartly each morning and heading out in heels and gloves to chase her career. The future brightened, until one fateful August morning just days into her new promotion. Little did Mona know that her dreams would soon crumble and plunge her into a fight for survival.

The Monster Called Polio

Mona awoke late that summer morning in 1956 full of anticipation for her job. As she dressed and fixed a quick breakfast, an unusually vicious headache brewed behind her eyes. She considered staying home, but stubborn persistence pushed her out the door. All morning the pounding in her skull intensified until light and sounds stabbed like knives at her brain. As she waited for the afternoon bus home, she realized she could barely stand. Somehow Mona managed the long trolley ride back to her apartment, waves of feverish nausea threatening to overtake her. She collapsed into bed, burrowing beneath blankets to shut out the excruciating pain ricocheting through her body.

Over the next two days, Mona careened between bouts of fever and increasing paralysis. Her aunt and uncle feared that death hovered at their door as she lay unresponsive for hours. Finally, her uncle bundled her limp body into his car racing to the hospital. Mona slipped in and out of consciousness, catching glimpses of white coats hovering as she was whisked into an exam room. She woke once more to urgent voices and realized a doctor stood over her holding critical lab reports. His words sliced through her stupor. "It's polio, a severe case. We may already be too late."

Over the preceding decades, summertime outbreaks of the highly contagious poliovirus decimated families across America. The disease attacked the central nervous system, often starting with flu-like stiffness that rapidly caused paralysis. In severe cases like

Mona's, the virus targeted motor neurons controlling muscles necessary for breathing. With no cure or treatment, physicians helplessly watched their young patients suffocate while hooked to primitive metal breathing aids. Though a vaccine introduced in 1955 promised hope, cases continued as the disease ran its course.

Now, at just 20 years old with most of her life ahead of her, Mona found herself a victim of the infamous scourge. As emergency staff rushed an iron lung to her bedside, she grasped the dire prognosis facing her. The monstrous device resembled a cylindrical metal coffin, big enough to encase her entire body up to the head. Fighting claustrophobic panic, she focused on each labored breath while doctors secured her inside. The iron lung enclosing her worked by changing air pressure to forcibly expand her paralyzed chest muscles. As the machine did the work of breathing for her, Mona finally relaxed into a much-needed sleep.

The next several months passed in a blur of agony as Mona fought the virus ravaging her body. The iron lung and medical interventions kept her alive but offered little relief from excruciating muscle spasms. She screamed herself hoarse from the pain, writhing against the unforgiving metal. When exhaustion finally granted a reprieve, she woke terrified that each breath might be her last. Doctors postulated that her robust health before contracting polio gave her a fighting chance, though they hesitated to make predictions. Paralyzed from the neck down, Mona could only watch helplessly as friends and family rallied around her.

Her parents rushed to Kansas City to join the hospital vigil, keeping watch through sleepless nights. Elmer paced the halls, face carved in worry over his once vibrant child now motionless in her metal coffin. Mary perched at Mona's bedside, stroking her fevered brow and humming comforting hymns. Mona drank in her mother's loving presence between random attacks.

She managed a weak smile when her high school
sweetheart Tom visited, though she turned away his
anguished attempts at affection. Between strenuous
breaths, she broke things off, unwilling to see pity
cloud his boyish devotion.

The darkest hours came as Mona wrestled internally
against the crippling damage. Angry screams gave way
to desperate prayers and finally quiet defeat. She
questioned what sin caused God's punishment in the
form of a deadly disease. The heart monitor registered
her despair as vital functions slowed dangerously low.
But as she lingered near death, a reserve of untapped
strength emerged; she chode to keep on fighting.
Mona stubbornly determined that giving up so soon
cheated fate of a greater destiny awaiting. She ordered
medical staff to continue aggressive treatments,
rallying her family to push through. If she regained
but a fraction of motion, she could salvage meaning
from her catastrophe.

Miraculously, after three months tethered to the iron lung, Mona stabilized. Doctors rejoiced as tingling and muscle twitches signaled the virus loosening its grip. Therapists gingerly helped her sit upright, though still relying on the metal exoskeleton for air-hungry lungs. After months of gazing at sterile ceilings, Mona wept at the beautiful sunset from her wheelchair. As autumn leaves drifted by the hospital window, everyone breathed easier regarding her survival. The long road of rehabilitation lay ahead, but there was hope.

Hard Won Recovery

Discharge papers in hand, Mona looked expectantly from the taxi to her little walkup apartment. But suddenly she hesitated. While she mastered breathing unassisted for several hours, nights still required the iron lung's mechanical assistance. Maneuvering the hulking device up three flights of narrow stairs seemed impossible. Noticing her panic, the volunteer attendant squeezed Mona's hand reassuringly before waving over a truck idling at the curb. Orderlies promptly loaded the iron lung onto a lift gate, hoisting it effortlessly to her front door. Mona bit her lip watching the scene, realization sinking that from now on, such elaborate arrangements preceded any outing. Her sunny apartment overlooking the park now needed retrofitting to accommodate her disability from weakened lungs. She must adapt her life to the medical apparatus instead of the other way around. Mona took a deep breath and turned her chair toward the ramp installed next to the front steps. She was grateful to be home again.

Over the next year, Mona settled into her new normal, strictly regimenting days to optimize limited energy. Mornings began the laborious process of getting up. Her helper cautiously hoisted her dead-weight limbs from the bed into the wheelchair. Breakfast required Mona to either be hand-fed or utilize her stiff arthritic fingers to painstakingly grasp a spoon that felt like it was bolted to the table.

She persevered through uncomfortable stretching sessions to keep atrophying muscles pliable. Though afternoons allowed a few glorious hours free of the iron lung, she monitored the clock to avoid crushing fatigue. Still, Mona stubbornly insisted on as much independence as her frail body allowed, telling her helpers to stand down while she struggled to dress and bathe alone. Only the simple mechanics of survival filled her days, yet she carved happiness from small triumphs over her limitations.

As weeks stretched into years, Mona gradually expanded her world once more. Her sister Martha provided a lifeline to normalcy, the two giggling like schoolgirls over coffee or debating world affairs. Mona welcomed close friends to small gatherings showing off new feats like feeding herself. During summers, a van taxi transported her to Lake Pomona just outside the city. There she could sit wheelchair-bound yet free, remembering what the wind in her hair felt like. Although polio robbed her limbs, it freed her mind to soar. She now voraciously consumed literature, history, and religion; quality knowledge to feed her restless intellect.

While sealed in her metal enclosure, several questions haunted Mona's restless nights. She knew she was extraordinarily lucky to be alive while neighbors and celebrities like FDR perished from the devastating illness. Why then did she linger in such debilitating limbo, too weak to fully participate in life yet denied ultimate peace? She worried polio's cruel trick sentenced her to forever fall short of her dreams. But a quote from a psychologist's lecture stirred a revelation; "luck was not random chance but opportunity meeting preparation." In her darkest valley, she committed to recovery so that when the door for more open, she could walk through without hesitation. The key was changing their perspective on life not serving her. Mona's spirit was renewed with the realization that meaning, purpose and even transformation grow from adversity. She resolved that however long she had; it would be lived abundantly by embracing new dreams.

Steps Toward Living a Purposeful Life

Eager for purpose, Mona enrolled in seminary classes at a local university. She soaked up lectures on ethics and listened raptly to theologians debate morality. Studying fueled introspection on divisive social issues and her responsibility to address injustice. She felt called to enact the charge "to whom much is given, much is required". Her struggle living with disability opened people's eyes to the lack of accessibility and inclusion in society. Having borne the yoke of oppression, she now felt bound to relieve others still trapped.

Mona's advocacy work began close to home with practical needs for the severely handicapped. Her injury cut short her professional aspirations to become self-sufficient, forcing reliance on family generosity. Many others with disabilities navigated dire financial straits, struggling to afford basic medical care. She partnered with state rehab organizations to sponsor job retraining and independent living programs. Training peer counselors provided both meaningful work and invaluable advice to the newly disabled. She rejoiced at the progress in securing handicapped employment protections in the 1964 Civil Rights Act.

Spurred by her aunt's wheelchair confinement from arthritis, Mona rallied city resources toward disability infrastructure reforms. At her urging, Kansas City transportation officials agreed to test curb cuts allowing wheelchair access. She helped draft accommodations guidelines adopted nationally guaranteeing accessibility in public state and federal buildings. Seeing tangible change emerge from her efforts reignited Mona's long-dormant aspirations. Though still tethered to the iron lung nightly, her relentless activism imprisoned no one.

A Spiritual Awakening

Mona's paralytic imprisonment forced her not to just advocate for others, it also gave her a deeper confrontation with her Christian faith. In seminary studies, she closely examined the doctrine about adversity either being punishment for sin or a redemptive form of suffering. But reconciling a supposedly just God with her debilitating affliction proved impossible. Her family, faith leaders, and even doctors sometimes blamed her paralysis on personal failings or cosmic retribution. Their prosperity gospel held that declaring healing by faith alone miraculously restored health.

Such facile explanations only amplified Mona's crisis of confidence in divine purpose. She fixated on scripture promises that through grace, the faithful could transcend infirmity. Had she not prayed fervently enough to make her paralyzed legs walk again? Cold logic concluded that either her prayers lacked conviction or God lacked power and will. As resentment and disbelief threatened to overwhelm her, she pleaded aloud for wisdom and comfort. Only stillness echoed back, exacerbating the sense that she was undeserving of a miracle. Mona nurtured secret certainty that she was being tested and found wanting.

The turning point came unexpectedly during a life-threatening medical crisis. Battling pneumonia, Mona struggled for each labored breath while fluid slowly filled her lungs. Without the strength to cough, she suffocated as monitors registered critically low oxygen levels. Certain that death approached, panic gripped her. Then suddenly, revelation-like understanding dawned that this moment presented a choice. She saw two divergent paths, either cling to anger at divine betrayal or fully surrender herself to God with absolute trust despite unanswered petitions. Without hesitation, she let go of resentment and fear. A profound peace enveloped her as she relinquished attempts to bargain on her terms. She simply rested in faith that her life and death served eternal purposes beyond understanding. She gave thanks for unexpected blessings because adversity nurtured this unquenchable joy and freedom.

Shortly after, almost miraculously, Mona began recovering from pneumonia. But of far greater importance was spiritual healing, the liberation of handing complete control to divine will. Polio's paralytic blow crushed more than just muscle and nerve; it externalized the infirmity of doubt dwelling within. Now Mona walked the path of humility accepting grace sufficient for weakness. She learned to separate useless lament over a broken body from celebrating the wholeness of purpose. Going forward, her sacred mission was aiding fellow travelers to live abundantly despite limitations. No longer defined by disability, she saw herself as an instrument to manifest holy truths.

Opening Doors for Others

Her newly energized spirit translated into renewed vigor advocating for Kansas City's disabled residents. Mona took a position consulting at the city's rehabilitation research training center. Their work pioneered independent living programs fostering self-sufficiency for handicapped citizens. Her insight proved invaluable in assisting quadriplegics and accident victims to regain dignity, if not mobility. She counseled new paraplegics on managing injury grief and channeling anger into empowerment. Drawing on her expertise in navigating inaccessibility, she guided architects in designing barrier-free housing. Mona even collaborated with engineers at NASA, testing concepts to help mobility-impaired astronauts remain professionally active. Each small breakthrough lifted the veil of helplessness that shrouded people with disabilities.

Mona also collaborated with local government agencies supporting those unable to work. She advocated for expanding social security disability programs providing both medical coverage and living stipends. Her testimony before legislative finance committees ensured adequate funding safeguards for Kansa's most vulnerable. Many people admitted dealing with disabilities only through intermediaries before meeting the vivacious Mona. Her fierce intelligence and savvy negotiation skills won over skeptics unused to seeing the severely handicapped as equals.

Despite her accomplishments so far, Mona still worried about the steady decline of her body, now threatening her hard-won independence. Weakened lungs left her relying ever more on mechanical breathing assistance. She often woke gasping and unable to trigger her device's automatic controls. Though committed staff helped transition her to bed each evening, no one could fully attend to her round the clock. She steadfastly refused relegation to a care facility despite pleas that her family could no longer cope alone.

The solution came from an unlikely place—her church community. Mona's mission of aiding disabled acquaintances fostered unlikely friendships, including several parishioners from Colonial Presbyterian. Inspired by her selfless example, Debbie and Warren Graham made a remarkable offer upon hearing her struggles. They proposed establishing a faith-based communal residence with live-in support tailored to Mona's needs. She would direct planning to prove that with problem-solving and compassion, ordinary people could provide extraordinary care. Their vision was so aligned with Mona's inclusive values that she tearfully accepted the proposal.

Mona named the residence Abounding Love to reflect the quality of care offered within. The accessible house accommodated both her breathing equipment and several caretaker bedrooms. With round-the-clock assistance guaranteed, Mona regained confidence leaving home daily without counting down to exhaustion.

She particularly cherished nightly gospel readings and hymns sung over her iron lung cocoon by her "family." For nearly 15 years, Mona led worship and outreach inspiring empathy for marginalized populations. Though many residents cycled through, most considered their stint at Abounding Love lifechanging. More than a few even entered healthcare fields or ministries due to her influence.

When unable to travel abroad for mission work, Mona directed efforts locally serving vulnerable groups. She educated her comfortable suburban church on the challenges confronting urban homeless and addict populations. Mona led fundraising for Colonial Presbyterian's food pantry and addiction counseling programs. She cofounded Abounding Love ministry which matched church members as mentors to children and adults with developmental disabilities. For once a month, her delight filled the building as clients and volunteers danced, played games, and broke bread together. Though disease continued eroding her physical functions, Mona's vibrant mind and generous heart elevated everyone she touched.

A Blessed Marriage

Incredibly, amidst the 24-hour care juggle of breathing machines, doctor visits, and advocacy work, Mona found love. She met Mark Randolph in her mid-40s through Colonial Presbyterian's widower grief support group. The church paired the recent widowers, hoping they could provide peer counsel. But immediately upon meeting, the two struck up a conversation that flowed for hours. The next week Mona invited Mark to help serve at Abounding Love dinner, wanting to showcase this passion in her life. Watching her in her element, joyfully connecting church and community members, filled him with immense respect. Though he assisted in transferring her in and out of the iron lung each evening, the machinery quickly faded behind her vibrant spirit.

Within months, their relationship shifted from mutual bereavement to an adoring partnership. Mona never expected marriage given the extreme confinement of her disability. But Mark delighted in slowly wooing her with poetry reading and handicap-accessible dates. When asking her elderly father for the blessing to propose, Elmer gruffly warned that caretaking would exhaust him. But glancing from Mark's earnest face to daughter's radiant smile, he smiled himself. "I

reckon you youngsters understand love ways I ain't
got words for," he conceded. At their small outdoor
wedding with the iron lung discretely parked beside
the arbor, joyful tears defined the start of a new
blessed season.

The storybook image of the older couple gazing
lovingly despite adversity captured media attention.
Feature profiles on local news and in newspaper
spreads focused on Mona as an iron lung "anomaly."
She fielded calls from across the country from other
polio survivors struggling with post-disease effects on
weakened muscles. As demand for her personal story
increased, she obliged interview requests to highlight
ongoing hardships faced by her community. Mona
candidly discussed construction to support 500
pounds of metal ambulance transported to speaking
events and overnight hotel stays. She gamely
demonstrated the intricate bedtime routine aided by
Mark and the nursing staff to settle into her yellow
submarine.

Privately Mona wrestled frustration over reduction to merely a medical oddity defined by equipment keeping her alive. Mark rubbed her shoulders consolingly as she vented annoyance at invasive questions on toileting and intimacy. Didn't decades tirelessly devoted to counseling, advocacy, and ministry merit focus too? Sensing this, Mark encouraged Mona to work with a writer to capture the full memoir she deserved. He dreamed a book might bring overdue respect, financial security, and widespread inspiration. Though initially hesitant to glorify hardship, Mona warmed to the idea of imparting hard-won wisdom. After gentle encouragement from her devoted husband, she committed fully to an autobiography project almost four decades disabled.

Mona spent several years filtering through her remarkable life to compile an eloquent narrative. Peeling back the long-repressed pain of descending into radical disability proved emotionally exhausting.

She wept hot tears at the magnitude of loss every time assistants lifted her limp legs. Yet she found catharsis thanking caretakers, doctors, and her younger self for persevering over impossible odds. Transcending physical and spiritual brokenness to arrive at purpose felt like both climax and benediction to closing this volume of her life.

Before the memoir reached its final draft, unexpected setbacks derailed their efforts. A bout of pneumonia left her fragile lungs less durable. Despite aggressive interventions, the damage scarred fragile tissues accelerating her decline. Virtually overnight Mona lost the ability to breathe without the iron lung, hastening round-the-clock assistance. Confident that the book conveyed her legacy sufficiently through this late chapter, she reluctantly set aside completing it for managing the final season with grace.

Mona coped steadfastly with intensifying immobility by focusing on beloved routines. Mark noted his once restless wanderer now rarely left the bedroom and adjacent sitting area. Her nurse transferred Mona there daily to enjoy the view outdoors through picture windows. Though every passing season allowed fewer hours sitting upright, she savored her favorite poetry books and hymns filling quiet days. Regular visits from her pastor and devoted husband kept loneliness at bay as her world condensed.

Mona's Final Moments

When too feeble to continue directing affairs, Mona entrusted Mark to manage her care decisions. She found great comfort in trusting her needs and now her life rested safely in his compassionate hands. Outside of occasional trip planning for the nursing staff, Mona permitted herself to stop chasing last wishes. Instead, she invested long peaceful moments gazing into his eyes to silently impart her heartfelt gratitude for the gift of partnership. She told Mark often that his stalwart love inspired her decades-long fight against all odds. Now at the end, she felt prepared to slip into whatever mystery followed, sustained by that love.

On a cold February evening, as Mark leaned down for their nightly kiss sealing the iron lung, Mona held him close for several heartbeats. Snow swirled outside framing them in ethereal light, the present moment crystallized into perfection. As Mark finally pulled away, a beatific smile graced her weary face. "Parting is such sweet sorrow dearest. I'll be watching for you," Mona whispered. Drawing a last gentle breath, she surrendered herself to eternal rest.

Mark tucked her favorite poetry book between clasped hands crossing her chest before finally closing the casket lid. He stood vigil until the ambulance arrived, irrevocably moved by witnessing a saint's tranquil passing. Randolph passed away on February 18, 2019, following complications from her condition.

In the decades since those blessed to be touched by Mona Jean Randolph carry precious fragments of her legacy forward. The organizations she spearheaded continue providing critical services to Kansas City's marginalized communities. From hospital wards to shelter kitchens, professionals frequently invoke guiding principles she enacted serving vulnerable populations. Several progressive policies improving accessibility and empowering the disabled emerged directly from her tireless activism.

But perhaps Mona's most enduring legacy breathes through the countless souls she shepherded from life's dark valleys back into the light. Though confined physically, her spirit soared free to encourage dreams beyond limits. The iron lung sustained her body yet circumscribed nothing, not her bold vision benefiting generations nor her transformational act of loving without restraint. Hers was a calling to manifest divine grace and, in that purpose, she continues reminding humanity that within brokenness often dwells beauty. Mona Randolph lived passionately by embracing each breath as a gift enough to change the world. Hers was a life triumphing abundance emerging even from adversity.

Chapter 8

Paul Richard Alexandra's Story

Paul Richard Alexander was born on January 30th, 1946 in Dallas, Texas. His early years were filled with joy and typical child's play. He would roam the suburban neighborhoods of north Dallas, playing tag in the streets with groups of lively children. Baseball in summer and exploring the woods in springtime were his frequent favorite pastimes. By all accounts, Paul was a normal American child leading an ordinary 1950s childhood.

That all changed abruptly in 1952 when at age six, Paul contracted polio, a disease that swept through towns nationwide crippling and killing thousands of young people annually. As with many children, Paul's parents watched helplessly as the energetic boy they loved rapidly declined for days marked by fevers, fatigue, and loss of appetite. Soon Paul lost all capacity for movement and autonomy. The poliovirus had irreparably damaged his motor neurons, leaving his muscles paralyzed and his lungs failing. Paul's entry into hospital isolation marked the end of his childhood innocence. What followed would permanently alter the trajectory of his life.

Surviving Against All Odds

During the peak polio years in America, infection meant likely death or lifelong confinement to restrictive metal respirators called iron lungs. As polio attacked the nerve cells controlling Paul's diaphragm and chest muscles, doctors rushed to connect the dying six-year-old to one of the dreaded iron tombs before he suffocated.

Initially able to tolerate only minutes at a time breathing independently, Paul lived encased up to his neck in the iron lung's airtight cylindrical chamber. Its automated bellows rhythmically expanded and compressed, mechanically drawing breath in and out of Paul's dormant lungs. This cycle continued around the clock, granting Paul borrowed time.

Death regularly surrounded Paul in the hospital polio ward. Kids in iron lungs frequently succumbed to the failure of overtaxed organs like the heart and kidneys. Of all children with paralytic polio, only 2 in 10 survived the first two weeks using iron lungs. Paul watched helplessly as nurses removed the bodies of children he befriended, kids robbed of futures as wives, artists, and fathers. Why God spared him but let others die never stopped haunting Paul's restless mind.

Reclaiming Life Outside the Iron Coffin

Though liberated from imminent suffocation by the iron lung, Paul refused to accept this as his ultimate destiny. He believed continuing existence must hold meaning if only he persevered to find it. With a firm determination Paul committed to regaining some independence, starting with the most basic yet elusive goal: learning to reliably breathe enough air without his respiration aid machine to permit some waking hours out of its clutches.

Paul enlisted the help of a sympathetic nurse who incentivized his training by promising a puppy if he could sustain three minutes of independent breathing. She coached him daily, expanding his lung capacity using specialized techniques requiring immense discipline and frustration tolerance. Progress was glacially slow, marked by frequent severe setbacks forcing Paul back into the iron lung.

Miraculously, after a year of intensive respiratory muscle conditioning, Paul could remain outside his mobile prison for three entire minutes before signals of oxygen deprivation mandated his return. With encouragement from his medical team, Paul increased his tolerable duration without mechanical breathing assistance first to thirty minutes, then to two hours.

This hard-fought success opened new worlds for Paul to conquer. No longer continuously tethered to the large, cumbersome machines that filled hospital rooms, Paul gained unprecedented mobility and freedom. His horizons expanded as he directed his electric wheelchair throughout hospital corridors. What once seemed impossible now appeared within reach through sheer determination.

Escaping Hospital Walls for University Halls

Indefatigable resolve led Paul to set his sights on lofty goals including finishing school studies interrupted when disease derailed his childhood. Knowing polio denied him physical access to traditional classrooms, Paul petitioned his local school board for a special exception granting him status as one of Texas' first home-schooled students.

Through diligent self-study with materials collected by devoted family members, Paul not only finished high school but was accepted to attend university while reliant on his iron lung. Southern Methodist University (SMU) became the first of several colleges Paul attended en route to an eventual law degree. Perhaps more impressive than Paul's academic feats was navigating university life while tethered to an antiquated 300-pound respirator.

To attend classes on campus Paul defied skeptics claiming such goals remained out of reach, instead moving himself and his aging iron lung into campus dorms alongside more typical students. With help from a shift of trained assistants, Paul shuttled to class wheeled in a gurney-mounted iron lung then transferred into a small mobile respirator for hours at a time. At night and whenever fatigue from breathing independently set in, he retreated to the relative safety of full enclosure back in his dorm. Jaws regularly dropped the first-time students and school staff saw Paul maneuvering through campus inside the Iron respirator.

A Lawyer in an Iron Lung

After excelling through his university studies, Paul set his sights on an even more unlikely professional aspiration; practicing law from inside his iron shell. Naysayers said managing unpredictable courtroom hearings without the capacity to take bathroom breaks or speak loudly enough to address juries remained beyond reasonable goals for someone requiring round-the-clock mechanical breathing support. As before, Paul ignored doubters.

After earning his Juris Doctor in 1984, Paul passed the bar exam on his first attempt. He soon opened his law practice, commuting to a local office suite. There, Paul made legal history as the vision of a man encased neck-deep in a hissing black bellows machine arguing cases. This shocked judges and opponents unfamiliar with his bizarre condition. With an alphabet board and skilled interpreter at his side, Paul ably advocated for clients. His disability lent an indelible underdog ethos that juries responded to favorably.

Later Years: Embracing Interdependence

Reaching his 70s, Paul requires ever greater support performing basic tasks like eating, washing, and adjusting his position in bed. Round-the-clock caregiving by assistants permits Paul to continue directing his affairs using voice commands and by mouthing words interpretable to the trained eyes of caregivers accustomed to translating his unique communications.

Though still frequently troubled at night by anxieties about the mechanical failure of aging equipment keeping him alive, Paul struggles against mindsets of helplessness. He believes fixating on fears and self-pity only serves to constrain the possibilities remaining to him. Instead, Paul focuses on directing caretakers regarding his needs and desires to make the most of each day on his terms. Though his body progressively fails him in new ways, Paul's intellect and adventurous spirit remain as resilient as ever.

The journey of Paul Richard Alexander provides a remarkable portrait of courage and perseverance in the face of immense human suffering. His willingness to endure discomfort and danger to author the life story he envisioned should inspire anyone facing daunting odds stacked to the neck against them. Anyone confronting loss and limitation can do well to follow Paul's lead. His incredible story puts on full display that circumstances beyond one's control need not overly determine life's richness or its capacity for purpose. By revealing the immense latent potential lying dormant within, Paul's astonishing path offers inspiration to people from all walks of life.

Chapter 9

Audrey J. King's Story

Audrey King was just nine years old when she contracted polio in 1952 while her family was living in England. Her father was in the army, stationed overseas, and Audrey remembers that fateful day when she first felt ill. She was taken to the hospital on a stretcher, staring up at the tiles on the ceiling as she was wheeled through the halls. After being settled into a room and hearing babies crying next door, Audrey made one last attempt to stand up before collapsing back onto the bed, her legs suddenly lifeless and limp.

The next day, Audrey found herself unable to breathe on her own. She has stark memories of being carried quickly into another room and placed inside a large wooden box; an iron lung. Audrey spent the next two days drifting in and out of consciousness, confused about what was happening but struck by a little China cup with a spout sitting on a windowsill behind her head. It was her first encounter with the apparatus that would sustain her breathing for the next two months.

The iron lung enveloped Audrey's entire body up to her head in an airtight chamber. A rubber collar was fastened snugly around her neck to seal the area. The other end of the long box was connected to a pump with bellows that would rhythmically suck the air out of the chamber. This caused Audrey's lungs to expand forcefully and pull in oxygen, essentially breathing for her since her diaphragm muscles were now paralyzed. Then the bellows would stop, allowing the chamber to fill up with air again before repeating the vacuum cycle. The resulting sound was like someone breathing loudly in and out at steady intervals.

Lying motionless in the isolated hospital room day after day, staring up at the tiled ceiling, Audrey struggled profoundly with boredom. To pass the time, she would imagine traveling along the wire trailing from the light switch up the wall and onto the ceiling, pretending she was bicycling through her village and mapping out landmarks in her mind. In the mirror angled above her head, Audrey could see clouds drifting by outside her window. She decided the white clouds must be heaven, and the ominous dark ones were where the devil lived.

Her parents were the only visitors allowed, so Audrey ached for her brother and friends whom she was unable to see. The isolation compounded her despair. Well-meaning adults would make insensitive comments within earshot about her being a burden or needing to live in a home by the sea. Audrey still feels guilty recalling the sadness her situation brought her mother. Many years later, reading her mother's diary from that period finally gave Audrey insight into how

terrified her parents were, believing the doctor when
he told them to prepare for her imminent death. The
phases of grief, heartache, fervent prayers, and
eventual miraculous hope that carried them through
were recorded in that journal.

To help her pass the time, Audrey received books from
her school and attentive gifts from friends. A neighbor
faithfully sent little glass animal figurines for her
collection. The two lady missionaries who visited
Audrey didn't realize they were fueling her childhood
crush when they brought her a stuffed black cat which
she named Herkimer Zebulon Picaro King. Their
good-natured laughter at her earnest jokes brought
only momentary embarrassment.

After two months encased in the iron lung, Audrey
was finally taken out and moved to a recovery bed.
The liberation was terrifying at first, constantly
panicking over whether she could breathe without

mechanical help. A nurse sat vigil that entire first night, ready to assist. What followed were years confined to hospitals, undergoing extensive therapy and rehabilitation to regain her natural body functions.

The adults marveled at cute little Audrey's pluckiness, but being so much younger than the other patients was isolating. A highlight in her early days was getting to participate in the Christmas festivities and broadcast from her hospital ward, feeling momentarily special instead of merely a sick child.

By age 11, Audrey had missed nearly six years of schooling. Periodic unsuccessful attempts to return to class convinced her local tutor that Audrey was unteachable. Finally, back home in Canada, her mother's assertive request secured Audrey's acceptance at the brand-new high school down the street. She credits the principal's open-minded willingness to make accommodations, combined with her schoolmates' help navigating the building, as giving her the first real sense of belonging and being like a regular student.

University brought more victories and milestones, leading to Audrey's rewarding 30-year career as a psychologist. That professional status and chance to make meaningful contributions to others' lives were pivotal in cementing her self-confidence and identity beyond disability.

Reflecting on her childhood, Audrey regrets the social isolation and lost the opportunity to have typical adolescent experiences. But she is grateful for her parents' resolute protection from situations that would have further damaged her self-image or exposed her weaknesses. The resilience Audrey continues exhibiting today is a testament to their unwavering love and faith in her potential.

Audrey's initial years back home in Canada were full of soaring accomplishments marred by periods of medical setbacks. She was thrilled at returning to school for a while at age 15 but was consistently stricken with new health problems that often confined her back at home.

One emotional blow came with the necessity of being put on the "cuirass ventilator" at night. Audrey describes it as an intermittent vacuum chamber sealing over her chest, rhythmically assisting with breathing while she slept by forcing her lungs to inhale. Where the old iron lung had encompassed her entire body, the cuirass felt less oppressive in some ways. But strapping on this artificial aid every night made her almost unbearably resentful after finally being free of the iron lung for five blessed years.

Audrey worried the cuirass would invite hurtful comments or questioning stares, making her feel embarrassed. Her ever-supportive parents rallied around her emotional needs yet again. They went on a camping trip that summer, towing a small trailer with all of Audrey's medical equipment inside. At the campsite, her father purchased hundreds of yards of extension cords at the hardware store to string electricity from the utility complex to their site, all so his daughter could have access to the power her cuirass ventilator required that night. His willingness to accommodate her needs gave Audrey courage and weakened her shame of over-relying on such unfamiliar devices.

In 1959, at age 19, Audrey enrolled at Queen's University in Ontario, Canada for her undergraduate degree. It was her first major separation from the constant support of her parents, and she approached this new phase anxiously yet eagerly. Having to advocate for herself more strenuously to receive appropriate accommodations awakened Audrey's resolve and bolstered her self-confidence.

Navigating the new experiences of campus life on her own tested Audrey sorely at times. Inadequate housing, insensitive roommates, inaccessible buildings, and classrooms, all posed obstacles she doggedly knocked down by speaking up assertively and appealing to authorities higher up for assistance when needed. Audrey credits the mentorship of certain compassionate professors as being instrumental in helping her acclimate.

Her psychology studies fed Audrey's fascination with human behavior and what motivates personal development. She earned excellent grades and impressed her professors by capably leading small classroom discussions with unique insights. During those sessions, Audrey often steered conversations towards thought-provoking analysis of how societal attitudes and language usage impact marginalized groups. Coursework on identity formation and overcoming adversity resonated with her profoundly.

Audrey lived frugally as a student to afford to hire daily personal attendants to assist with dressing, errands, meal preparation and generally navigating a world not designed for wheelchair users. Her zeal and charm eased her solitude and prevented her from experiencing total social isolation like she experienced growing up. Audrey intentionally positioned her attendants' chairs directly beside her wheelchair at campus events to participate more fully, rather than relegating them to the caregiver's role of hovering silently in the background per custom. She appreciated their friendship enormously.

In 1963, Audrey graduated magna cum laude with her Bachelor of Arts degree in Psychology. She had defied others' low expectations at every turn through her hard work. Now, Audrey looked ahead eagerly to what career doors this fresh accomplishment might open to her.

After graduating from university, Audrey was determined to secure meaningful employment that would allow her to give back and make a difference in her community. However, job prospects for wheelchair users were incredibly limited in the early 1960s, regardless of impressive credentials. Even positions that seemed well-suited to someone with mobility impairments often failed at providing necessary accommodations once hired, quickly terminating disabled employees deemed more trouble than they were worth.

Audrey spent months submitting applications and interviewing before finally being offered a role as a vocational counselor at a rehabilitation facility for disabled youth. She recognized firsthand how invaluable it was to receive encouragement from someone who intimately understood the obstacles they faced. Audrey mentored the teens on setting realistic goals, problem-solving transportation logistics in advance, requesting workplace modifications early on, and disclosing only necessary medical details with employers.

Within her first year, Audrey had successfully placed over two dozen young people into fulfilling jobs that matched their interests and abilities. Her compassionate guidance equipped them to advocate for themselves by asking for help when needed on the job without allowing reliance on others to impede their work performance. Colleagues marveled at the way students blossomed under Audrey's coaching, gaining confidence to attempt tasks long deemed impossible.

In 1965, Audrey relocated to a children's rehabilitation hospital in Toronto to accept the position of Staff Psychologist assisting families of youth newly diagnosed with spinal cord injuries or disease progression resulting in disability. Drawing heavily on her own childhood experiences, Audrey worked one-on-one and led group sessions for both the patients and their parents. She provided counseling on the grief and adjustment process as well as coaching them in effective advocacy tactics when encountering barriers to community participation.

Audrey pursued night classes to obtain her Master's degree in Social Work over the next several years while continuing at the rehab hospital full-time. She wrote her thesis on improving transitional services for disabled young people aging out of pediatric facilities, a topic she was extremely passionate about. Audrey had painfully endured losing trusted doctors and caregivers herself upon turning eighteen and being abruptly forced into the adults-only healthcare system. Through surveying former patients, Audrey's research quantified the challenges around securing new specialists, equipment funding delays, provider education gaps in treating adults with childhood-onset conditions, and general feelings of devastation facing these young people.

Armed with two advanced degrees and a decade of relatable lived experience, Audrey became the supportive mentor she had desperately needed but never found as a teen. Her impact rapidly multiplied as she took on leadership roles at the rehab hospital while maintaining a reduced counseling caseload. Audrey led workshops at national conferences, contributed chapters to medical textbooks, and consulted at facilities across Canada on improving care transitions. She served on hospital boards and government committees crafting disability legislation, leveraged connections with prominent figures to fund special projects, and continued shining light on the overlooked needs of the people she had dedicated her life to serving.

In 1972, Audrey King's advocacy achievements were honored with the prestigious Canada Centennial Medal for service to her country. At just 32 years old, her trailblazing work had made sweeping ripples across society already. As she graciously accepted the award, Audrey hoped her rebellious teenage self could look proudly forward from the past at what unexpected joys the years held in store.

Through the 1970s, Audrey split her time between counseling pediatric patients, developing programs and partnerships to address major service gaps, and serving as an unrelenting voice demanding policy reform around disability rights issues. She testified passionately at government hearings and protests over inaccessible transit, adaptive equipment funding, workplace discrimination, and disability stereotyping in the media, unafraid to directly challenge powerful hospital administrators and political leaders. Where other activists relied on emotional appeals primarily, Audrey's calm expertise and irrefutable personal experiences gave her instant credibility and gravitas.

Behind the scenes, Audrey mentored the next generation of young disabled professionals entering the workplace, drawing on the lessons that served her so well. She reminded them to request accommodations unapologetically, ignore colleagues urging them to 'not make waves,' and leverage small workplace successes into progressively more influence. Audrey encouraged each one to recognize their latent leadership abilities waiting to be awakened. Her greatest pride was witnessing their bold advocacy taking shape.

Audrey married her devoted husband Paul in 1975 at age 35. They had met a few years prior at a fundraiser Audrey organized when Paul generously offered his public relations skills to promote the event. Having pursued her career wholeheartedly for so long before considering romance, their relationship unfolded gradually out of deep friendship and mutual respect.

Paul embraced every facet of Audrey's remarkable life with awe and admiration rather than trepidation. He cheerfully adapted their home to be wheelchair-accessible, helped review her speeches, traveled alongside Audrey to conferences, spent weekends working by her side on special projects for the hospital, and made all her passions his own. Their partnership only amplified Audrey's juggernaut efforts.

The 1980s accelerated Audrey's leadership influence exponentially. She cultivated relationships with international advocacy groups and rehabilitation programs serving developing countries, collaborating to bring specialized training across language and cultural barriers. Audrey's ground-breaking work establishing peer support networks and independent living centers became the model for communities world-wide seeking to shift away from institutionalization towards empowering those with disabilities to control their own lives.

Invitations for Audrey to present her programs in person took the couple on whirlwind trips across several continents throughout the decade. Each place they visited; Audrey was touched by the lines of young people in wheelchairs awaiting a chance to meet their heroine in person. She returned home more motivated than ever to tear down restrictions.

After thirty years with the pediatric rehab hospital, Audrey formally retired in 1995 at the age of 55 though maintaining involvement as Director Emeritus. Her reflections from decades as both counselor and champion left her overwhelmingly proud of how far things had transformed since her dehumanizing childhood hospitalizations. Witnessing kids, she first met as terrified young patients now flourishing as independent adults with families of their own brought Audrey profound joy. She had conquered spectacular heights indeed from such humble beginnings no one could have imagined.

Audrey embraced retirement's slower pace as an opportunity to focus energy on cherished personal passions set aside for decades due to her unrelenting career. Always an avid reader, she dove enthusiastically into book club discussions, competed in literature trivia tournaments, and began serving on the board of trustees for the local library system.

Having never learned many domestic skills growing up in medical facilities and then assisted by caregivers as an adult, Audrey enrolled in adapted cooking and gardening classes through an area nonprofit. Their grants supplied customized appliances allowing her to prepare meals independently alongside others using wheelchairs and limb differences. Audrey delighted in hosting elaborate dinner parties to show off new recipes mastered under the patient guidance of her teachers.

She likewise discovered a profound love of nurturing living things in the greenhouse program creating accessible gardening spaces with customized tables, pots, and tools accommodating diverse mobility needs. Laboring among friends to plant seeds and then celebrating the emergence of each perfect new blossom fulfilled Audrey's long-held desire to participate more actively in this beautiful rite of spring she had only ever previously observed passively.

As an empty-nester finally, with time to indulge in hobbies, Audrey made up for lost years by throwing herself wholeheartedly into various crafting classes too. She learned origami, quilt-making, candle-wicking, enameling jewelry, ceramic painting, and more. Audrey gifted elaborate handmade birthday and holiday presents with immense satisfaction, continuing to build eye-hand coordination that eluded her as a child when therapies focused almost exclusively on physical function to the exclusion of creative play.

Paul fully retired several years after Audrey so they were both available to dotingly welcome grandbabies into the growing family dynasty bearing the King's legacy. Being a Granny brought Audrey indescribable joy. She loved having infants and toddlers sit on her lap, taking little hands in hers while guiding their tiny fingers across Braille story pages then applauding exuberantly at each new word decoded. Audrey made certain her wheelchair-height kitchenette in the corner of the living room was always stocked with tasty snacks and beverages so preschoolers could "cook" whenever they came over.

When reading classic fairy tales with her granddaughters, Audrey playfully cast herself as the wise elder queen or village healer- going on thrilling adventures alongside princesses and woodland creatures. Her elaborately embellished accounts wove tender life lessons into every tale, affirming the children's self-worth and cultivating empathy. Audrey addressed disability openly, integrating matter-of-fact positive portrayals into her stories instead of dodging uncomfortable topics as previous generations tended to. She knew firsthand the dangers of raising kids who although able-bodied remain ignorant and insensitive to common differences.

As her older grandchildren became teens and young adults, Audrey made herself available as a trusted confidante—just like always. Listening without judgment, communicating unconditional love, and gently imparting wisdom formed the bedrock of Grandma Audrey's relationship with each one. She attended every extracurricular event possible, volunteered as an assistant coach for wheelchair sports teams when needed, and never failed to send each child affirming notes reminding them they were cherished.

When Audrey's first two grandchildren graduated college and embarked on careers in helping professions, no one who knew her well was surprised in the slightest. As Audrey sailed blissfully through her late 70s, she continued prioritizing precious time with both her local and overseas grandchildren flourishing into compassionate world-changers themselves. Never one to slow down despite advancing age, Audrey remained actively engaged supporting numerous disability charities and youth development programs she held dear.

She particularly loved serving as a mentor for teen girls of all abilities, using her childhood challenges around self-confidence and social skills as a gateway to deep bonding. With her trademark humor and grace, Audrey taught them to nurture self-acceptance, tune out unrealistic messaging from media, set ambitious goals unconstrained by societal barriers, and speak up unflinchingly to defend not only their rights but also those who lack an equal voice.

Her protégées frequently credited wise Grandma Audrey as the sounding board who helped them navigate pivotal life decisions. They would drive for hours just to curl up in her lap once more, breathing in the faint scent of lavender soap and listening to her steady breathing in the quiet. Being reminded of their intrinsic worth and potential through her gentle words untangled knots of anxiety and uncertainty. Audrey's comforting support had a truly magical power transporting these young ladies back into the carefree joy of pigtailed little girls they once were under her loving guidance.

Into her eighth decade, Audrey maintained a packed schedule of speaking engagements at universities and conferences focused primarily on cultivating the next generation's disability rights leaders. Student groups constantly competed to have her serve as the distinguished guest lecturer for diversity awareness events on their campuses because Mrs. King's authenticity gripped the young audience instantly.

Without fail, Audrey would wheel herself boldly to the very edge of the stage and then begin building rapport before diving into heavier content. Her signature opening involved scanning the crowded auditorium and asking students to raise their hands if they knew someone with a disability. As virtually every arm slowly lifted, Audrey would nod vigorously and declare this honest dialogue long overdue. The cheers swelled as she described her intent to move past pleasantries towards a more raw, transformative conversation about confronting ableism.

During the audience Q&A segments after her talks, a long line inevitably formed at the standing microphones snaking up side aisles. Impatient latecomers grumbled towards the back over being closed out of submitting questions before Mrs. King had to conclude. Attendees walked away inspired that evening but even more enthusiastic recipients were the student volunteers getting to interact with their esteemed guests one-on-one behind the scenes.

Without cameras capturing her every word for posterity now, Audrey dispensed priceless nuggets of wisdom to these emerging leaders as they discussed shared struggles authentically between just a few of them backstage. The disciples gathered closely around Audrey's wheelchair to strategize how best to apply her advice on their campuses. She always urged them to start small with what they could personally impact immediately. Her mantra echoed that changing society required devotion and persistence rather than grand performances. Plant seeds of truth; nourish respect in your sphere of influence. Progress flows outward in unexpected ways from there.

Chapter 10

Thomas Fetterman's Story

On a sunny autumn day in November 1953, eight-year-old Thomas Fetterman was running races in the schoolyard with his friends, laughing and soaking in the cheerful glow of childhood innocence. But suddenly, little Thomas kept stumbling and falling unexpectedly. He felt sharp waves of pain shooting through his head as if someone were pounding his skull with a hammer. His worried mother swiftly picked him up from school and brought him home, tucking the boy into bed. However, lifting even his head caused unbearable pain to shoot through Thomas's small body. Sensing something was wrong, his parents urgently called their trusted family physician Dr. Walters to examine the ailing child.

Upon close inspection, Dr. Walters suspected Thomas had developed a severe viral illness known as "the grippe," or influenza. He reassured the anxious parents that Thomas simply needed rest and fluids, prescribing him medications for the fever and body aches. But over the next few days, young Thomas only grew increasingly ill, with frightening new symptoms arising by the hour. He began struggling greatly with his breathing, feeling as if a heavy stone was compressing his chest. Thomas also lost his appetite entirely, while unquenchable thirst and waves of agony continually wracked his body without relief.

Seeing their beloved son's health rapidly deteriorating before their eyes, Thomas's parents decided to rush him to the emergency room at Hahnemann University Hospital in downtown Philadelphia. Doctors feverishly ran a series of tests on Thomas's failing body, trying to diagnose this mysterious illness attacking a once vibrant, healthy child. Their leading suspicion was now spinal meningitis, an infection of the membranes surrounding the brain and spinal cord that could turn deadly without swift treatment. Though a spinal tap test came back inconclusive, physicians began aggressively pumping Thomas with intravenous antibiotics, delivering rounds of excruciating penicillin injections directly into his muscles every two hours, day and night.

Too ill to even cry out in pain anymore, Thomas felt himself progressively fading away as the antibiotics failed to improve his condition. Then one day, overcome by crippling thirst, he instinctively dragged his frail body out of bed to reach the bathroom sink for water. But as soon as Thomas's feet hit the cold tile floor, both legs instantly collapsed under the weight of his slender frame, leaving the small boy helplessly sprawled across the hospital room floor. When nurses found him on their next check-in rounds, doctors raced to run another analysis of spinal fluid and bloodwork. This time, they sorrowfully discovered the culprit ravaging Thomas's body: polio. Also known as poliomyelitis or infantile paralysis, this highly infectious and incurable viral disease targets the nervous system, often causing irreversible paralysis. Philadelphia fell within the epicenter of outbreak hotspots during the last great polio epidemic that terrorized American families in the late 1940s-50s. And now, little Thomas had become its latest victim.

With Thomas confirmed to be actively shedding live poliovirus and at risk of infecting other vulnerable patients, he received orders to immediately transfer from Hahnemann Hospital over to a quarantined isolation ward at Montgomery Hospital in nearby Norristown borough. Thomas's parents trailed behind the ambulance in despair, forced to stand outside their son's new glass room while garbed in gowns and masks. Gazing at his ghostly pale figure encased behind the soundproof glass, Thomas's mother wept knowing that she could not even hold her baby's hand to comfort him in what could be his final moments. Adding further anguish, the hospital demanded all of

Thomas's personal belongings be surrendered and incinerated; clothes, books, and toys, to avoid spreading contaminants. He truly had nothing left except the hospital gown on his back.

At this point, Thomas's entire body had already become completely paralyzed by the poliovirus attacking his nervous system and shutting off communication between his muscles and brain. He described the sensation akin to experiencing full-body rigor mortis, unable to lift his head, shift his limbs, or even wiggle a single toe. He felt himself transforming into a helpless prisoner trapped within what now seemed like an alien shell rather than a body. Thomas stared aimlessly up at the isolation room ceiling day and night, with death hovering right within reach. He feared he would stop breathing at any second as the virus choked off control over the muscles enabling that life-sustaining function. This eight-year-old boy grappled with his mortality far sooner than any child should, realizing with sudden acuity how fragile yet precious life could be.

The isolation ward nurses attentively monitored Thomas's worsening respiratory distress around-the-clock. His polio-paralyzed chest muscles struggled intensely to expand his rib cage for inhaling and deflating his lungs to exhale. Things took a sharp turn when Thomas began losing his battle to keep breathing on his own. Doctors hurriedly transported him into an iron lung machine designed as intensive life support for critical polio patients experiencing total respiratory failure.

This large metal sarcophagus continuously pumped air in and out of Thomas's lungs via alternating pressure levels within the chamber. He would be sealed inside through a hole for his neck, while the iron lung essentially breathed for him through mechanically assisted pressure changes. During initial adjustment, Thomas admittedly found the bizarre whooshing and suction noises emitted by the iron lung strangely soothing once he got accustomed to the rhythm. The machine's reliable automation served as proof-of-life, reassuring him with every simulated inhale and exhale that he had not yet succumbed. He managed brief stretches of sleep between episodes of waking panic whenever his mind would race thinking of being forever trapped immobile inside this artificial respirator, completely void of independence and dignity.

What miraculously kept Thomas's hopes up was befriending an equally ill yet spirited middle-aged woman lying in the neighboring iron lung. She sustained partial paralysis below the waist but still retained strength in her arms and ability to speak clearly. This warm maternal figure not only watched over little Thomas like a guardian angel but displayed such grace and optimism in facing her tribulations. Despite imprisonment inside an impersonal life-support machine, this loving mother found contentment passing hours talking to her husband and three young kids who visited daily without fail. Witnessing their visible affection and commitment offered a flicker of light piercing through Thomas's engulfing darkness, a reminder that life pulsated forward even amid adversity. Her stalwart positivity proved contagious. Thomas felt profoundly grateful that this compassionate soul was accompanying him through the storm.

After enduring two long weeks of breathing via the coffin-like iron lung, Thomas's condition finally stabilized enough to wean off full-time mechanical ventilation. He underwent transfer to Sacred Heart Hospital's rehabilitation wing for recovering polio patients requiring lengthy aftercare. Thomas occupied a room alongside his new friend Wesley Davis, another eight-year-old boy paralyzed by polio who hailed from the same hometown just north of Philadelphia. Their instant rapport and shared boyhood mischievousness infused a sense of normalcy into hospital life, offering temporary respite from grim reality. During fleeting interludes of childhood frolicking when Wesley and Thomas managed to sneak off, they would take elevators upstairs to the hospital lab just for excitement feeding caged monkeys. Or some days a nurse might take pity and escort the stir-crazy boys outside on impromptu field trips to replenish depleted spirits, like special visits arranged to the small Norristown Zoo.

However, any illusion of normalcy evaporated when it was time for rehab sessions. Thomas endured exhausting twice-daily physical therapy utilizing the acclaimed Sister Kenny Method for polio aftercare. Nurses began by wrapping Thomas's full body in painfully scalding wool blankets, aiming to warm and loosen his stiff, contracted muscles and joints before manipulations. Sweet Miss Van Horn, Thomas's primary therapist, then manually stretched his limbs into agonizing contortions far beyond comfort.

Although very painful, this was the only way to gradually coax muscle movement and preserve flexibility. Bloodcurdling screams echoing from the rehab gym served as the soundtrack to their grueling days recovering motor function inch by inch.

The nuns also custom-fabricated leg braces enabling Thomas to practice walking between parallel bars while relying on crutches for support and balance. Gradually through grit and perseverance, feelings returned to Thomas's legs. After months of re-training muscle patterns to reactivate those dormant limbs, Thomas reached a pivotal milestone when the Sisters finally deemed him ready for mobility without the aid of braces. Nurse Annie and Sister Mary Margaret escorted an anxious Thomas into a padded gym room for his first wobbling attempts at crutch-walking. Thomas felt immense pride conquering those early triumphant steps crossing the room himself, which soon gave way to shock when the seemingly sweet nuns began sneakily kicking crutches out from under him to deliberately send poor Thomas crashing down onto the mats. This favorite nun pastime known as "teaching him how to fall" recurred daily much to Thomas's chagrin.

But he progressed quicker than anyone anticipated until Thomas could adeptly navigate stairs and most terrains. His upper body and core strength saw dramatic growth from the intensive mobility re-training as well. Thomas began tackling steps more swiftly and with ease than some of his non-disabled classmates when he later returned to school. Sister Annie Louise pulled Thomas aside after prayer one evening to bestow hand-carved wooden crutches as a graduation gift, which he cherished and continued using for decades to come. While saying farewell to hospital staff who felt like family after nearly a year's stay, Thomas carried the lessons learned about perseverance and human resilience forward into the next vital chapter ahead.

Throughout the agonizing months little Thomas spent hospitalized battling paralytic polio, his parents displayed incredible strength and devotion staying by their ailing son's side every step of the way. Thomas's childhood home situated nearly 50 minutes distance from the hospital still did not deter his dedicated mother and father from visiting him daily without fail, despite relying solely on public transportation.

Once when a disastrous double flat tire prevented his parent's scheduled hospital trip, they frantically telephoned the front nurse's station profusely apologizing for the unforeseeable delay, fretting over their son feeling abandoned. Though perhaps secretly appreciating one welcomed afternoon of solitude and rest from well-meaning parents perpetually fussing over him, Thomas deeply valued their loyal involvement during this traumatic period made more bearable by family support.

Beyond his immediate family's aid, an entire community banded together to raise Thomas's spirits and speed his recovery. Well-wishing friends from church and school handmade Get Well Soon cards delivering loving notes, while others stopping by Thomas's hospital room entertained him with comic books or puzzles for distraction. Generous neighbors even donated handcrafted toys for amusement like a miniature train boxcar with working wheels fabricated from pennies and dimes glued along the sides. Their thoughtful relief efforts reinforced to Thomas this powerful truth; that people can astound through immense goodwill and kindness even amid trying times when humanity's light threatens dimming.

After being separated from normal childhood and home for nearly twelve long months, Thomas finally earned discharge from the hospital to continue convalescing back at his parents' row house. Doctors encouraged him to return to school immediately and resume socializing with kids his age rather than enduring further isolation. The school unfortunately lacked any accommodations like wheelchair ramps for accessibility. Thomas's principal Mr. Roy and cleric Father Bartholomew decided to keep Thomas with his original class and peers superseded logistics or special arrangements for navigating stairs.

After missing an entire academic year battling polio, Thomas bravely returned despite the school still expecting a disabled student to ascend stairs independently without any structural modifications like ramps. Teachers allowed Thomas early dismissal between classes to clunkily manage each set of imposing steps one painful lunge at a time. He began sitting down and scooting up each riser on his bottom, hoisting both legs manually step-by-step while lugging crutches along. Sluggish and sweaty by the journey's end, Thomas made it to homeroom just as the late bell rang and the next lesson commenced. But within mere weeks Thomas no longer needed those patronizing head starts to labor up the stairs slowly.

His strengthening athletic upper body quickly
mastered agilely climbing steps two at a time!

While Thomas felt elated to reunite with familiar faces
and reclaim a welcome sense of normalcy, the
landscape had certainly shifted after everything he
endured. His grade-school peers now viewed Thomas
as an alien in their world, a sickly boy turned town
celebrity. Everyone knew Thomas as "the kid who got
polio;" a tragic anomaly garnering undue attention
relative to his actual popularity before falling famous
due to disease. Rather than coddling from newfound
notoriety due to his grit battling back from death's
door, Thomas encountered resentment and bullying
from lesser mature classmates. They envied the doting
sympathy he received, jealously adding salt to
wounds. "Fake limping" impersonations and getting
tripped in the hallway proved common provocations.

One small silver lining from Thomas's polio misfortune was gaining common ground with upperclassman Jonas Salk once news spread about his involvement in pioneering a radical medical miracle—the polio vaccine. The year Thomas fell devastatingly ill from polio—1952 ranked among the United States' absolute worst outbreaks on record, with nearly 60,000 children infected and over 3,000 deaths. While battling through recovery's arduous gauntlet himself in hospital isolation, Dr. Jonas Salk became a household name after successfully testing history's first anti-polio immunization. As a shining emblem of scientific promise symbolizing Thomas's emancipation from the disease, he held Dr. Jonas Salk in the highest celebrity esteem.

Thomas avidly followed news coverage of Dr. Salk's heralded "killed virus" polio vaccine through every trial, failure, and tweak until authorities finally sanctioned widespread public adoption in 1955; the year he returned to school. When their paths first crossed shortly after in the hallway, Thomas worked up the courage to approach his idol, Salk. He conveyed boundless admiration and gratitude for this visionary doctor's efforts to eradicate such a cruel disease that nearly killed Thomas and crippled tens of thousands of children annually. The famous Dr. Jonas Salk displayed kind graciousness while indulging his enthusiastic fans' burning inquiries about how the famed sugar cube vaccine gets manufactured. Thomas confided lingering anxiety about polio relapse potential, to which Salk comfortingly cited "less than one in a million odds." Without hesitation, Thomas voluntarily enrolled among the first eager recipients queued to receive Dr. Jonas Salk's celebrated polio immunization upon its initial 1955 Philadelphia school launch, safeguarding him from ever enduring that trauma again.

Another milestone deeply imprinted on Thomas's memory was witnessing the debut adventures of a fictional American TV folk hero that uniquely mirrored aspects of his youthful battle with adversity - Davey Crockett. This Disney dramatized miniseries starring the renowned actor Fess Parker broadcast shortly after Thomas's 1955 homecoming became an overnight national sensation, boosted by the title character's trademark raccoon fur cap sparking a popular fashion craze. Despite Thomas's original furry Davey Crockett hat purchased pre-polio perishing in the hospital incinerator, he harbored no bitterness. Even deprived of a signature cap like other boys that fad year, merely watching the King of the Wild Frontier's heroic portrayals on television transported Thomas on imaginative adventures transcending physical limitations.

Decades passed onward from the bittersweet year 1955 that saw Thomas tasting hard-earned autonomy again after enduring two crippling years battling polio's ruthless assault on his body. He entered adulthood still relying upon crutches and leg braces as mobility aids stemming from irreversible nerve and muscular damage. But defiantly refusing to let lingering disabilities dampen his indomitable spirit, Thomas devoted himself to experiencing full immersive life on his liberating terms without constraints. Setting ambitious global travel goals not typically attained by the able-bodied population either, Thomas boldly ventured halfway across the world backpacking extensively through India and Indonesia throughout months-long expeditions during the 1970s solo and with his loyal bride Cate by his side.

On one such trip passing through Santa Barbara where television's iconic 1950s frontier hero Davey Crockett retired into the hospitality business post-acting, Thomas decided to pay searching respects regarding that long-departed relic from his childhood. He gleefully spotted the now silver-haired Fess Parker proprietor emerging from his hotel lobby and could not resist harmonizing the nostalgic Davey Crockett theme song while limping on crutches toward the

Hollywood star stunned in recognition. Fess Parker amiably played right along, indulging their heartwarming reunion by finishing verses of the classic ditty rotating on transistor radios when they originally crossed paths through fate's TV screen portal. Upon hearing Thomas's poignant story of once dearly missing that symbolic raccoon cap destroyed by tragedy, his newfound friend Fess Parker voluntarily bestowed Thomas a replacement keepsake treasure as a touching gesture of camaraderie, a duplicate costume hat signed "To My Pal Thomas" hand-gifted from one resilient fellow adventurer to another!

Now facing the sixth decade of life travels relying upon carved crutches as mobility aids enabling greater autonomy than nature otherwise afforded, Thomas could no longer ignore the steep toll enduring years of mechanical stress had inflicted on his upper body. The necessary exertion demanded maintaining ambulation through wrist-joint support placed him at severe risk for early-onset arthritis and possible surgery. But rather than succumb to adversity or stagnate from despair, Thomas once more decided to embrace escalated hardship by devising creative solutions advancing not just self-preservation, but a launchpad for easing universal struggles shared by expanding communities.

Drawing from a lifelong affinity for tinkering with mechanical contraptions initially nurtured as a handicapped child concocting elaborately rigged toy trains, Thomas commenced work on customized crutch accessory prototypes aimed at minimizing sustained user joint damage through corrective alignment and buffering impact. After vigorously testing countless crutch tip mockup variations over consecutive years, Thomas ultimately engineered an ergonomically enhanced shock-absorbing crutch tip model superior to primitive hospital-issued options that had scarcely evolved since the Salk vaccine era. Once satisfied with performance safety metrics on his radical crutch tip design fortified with protective padding and angular swing joint, Thomas diligently secured official patent registrations followed by contracts with major health supply corporations. His uniquely intuitive mobility device invention born from necessity's workshop soon exceeded sales of 1 million units internationally, offered as standard durable medical equipment covered through insurance subsidies and VA disability provisions.

Word of this revolutionary crutch tip innovation gradually permeated global disability networks as Thomas' personalized brainchild benefiting countless fellow mobility aid users gained medical mainstream legitimacy. As an unexpected bonus, the mass distribution and consistent sale royalties from his patented ergonomic crutch tips proved rather lucrative over two decades as an accidental entrepreneur. Though never setting out originally seeking fortunes or fame, Thomas achieved both uniquely impacting lives for the better simply by creatively problem-solving his disability dilemmas.

This quintessential bootstrap journey from childhood misfortunes to a profitable industry pioneer profoundly enriches not just Thomas's story, but our civilization's larger narrative advancing empowerment for marginalized people.

Now a respected authority within international adaptive rehabilitation circles from trailblazing mobility device upgrades simple yet revolutionary, Thomas continually encounters the spectrum of crutch-dependent patients his designs liberate from unnecessary hardship. Each interaction with folks benefiting directly through his purposeful invention reminds Thomas precisely why shouldering the rigors battling his business concept from drawing board blueprint to store shelf fruition proved worthwhile. Every grateful testimony received from a stranger detailing how his crutch tips changed their life indelibly reaffirms the significance behind Thomas's unwavering perseverance.

When reflecting over six decades of living as a person with a disability, Thomas assesses contracting paralytic polio at the dawn of childhood proved one of the absolute best occurrences directing his life's upside trajectory, this shocking statement for sure given rational fears of contagious terminal illness. Were nature allowed to run its course uninterrupted, Thomas believes he may never have nurtured such grit, thankfulness, interdependence, ingenuity, or a sense of daring adventure distinguishing his rich life's resume from conceivably more ordinary outcomes. The resilience muscle polio forced him toning so early and extremely doubtlessly prepared Thomas to handle all subsequent adversity with staunch optimism and creative determination instead of defeatist despair.

Thomas's fulfilling family life as a devoted husband and father is certainly traced to securing a sizeable inheritance from surviving trauma and the maturation process. For example, he learned to instill confidence for independence rather than coddling overprotection from Cate; his wife possessing enough fiery grit for their whole clan. Also, Thomas treasures his bright grown daughter and baby granddaughter as his most cherished blessings. Yet poignantly watching his little grandbaby girl rapidly reach milestones of sitting, crawling, pulling ups, first tipsily brave steps gingerly taken, ultimately solo strolls trouncing everywhere with carefree innocence...Thomas profoundly appreciates life's fleeting beauty as only someone acquainted intimately with loss of function could. No moment gets taken for granted.

Even beyond immediate family though, the global community of fellow disabled persons Thomas discovered through shared empathy and struggle proved an unexpected gift sprouting from boyhood affliction. After selling a millionth patented crutch tip fast approaching 2025, Thomas could retire wealthy having never profited from medical merchandise before fate intervened. Crossing age 70, Thomas maintains passionate engagement supporting this beloved community of disabled people as an elder statesman passing torches to advise the next generations. Because the polio survivor network welcomed a scared hospitalized child without prejudice into their fold when Thomas needed belonging most, he dedicated himself to paying kindness forward.

No matter what unknown chapters or increasing twilight years ahead may reveal, Thomas knows contentment. Not ephemeral surface pleasures, but the abiding sort weathering storms. Thomas squeezed satisfactory living from adversity's very teeth despite his limitations. He sees the blessings granted to him now numbering 8 decades by experiencing so young how instantly Anyone's charmed routine existence could shatter overnight. With the privilege of perspective, Thomas understands why fearless optimism framing each sunrise feels fitting. This polio fighter won his battle long ago; henceforth each additional rising day feels nothing less than pure victory.

Chapter 11

Dianne Odell's Story

Dianne Odell spent nearly 60 years of her life encased in a 750-pound iron lung that enabled her to breathe. Though the machine severely restricted her movement and kept her confined to her home, Dianne lived a remarkably full life filled with education, writing, faith, and connection with others.

Dianne's Early Life

Dianne Freeman Odell was born on February 13, 1947, in Jackson, Tennessee to Freeman and Geneva Odell. She was the Odell's first and only child. Dianne's first few years were typical for the late 1940s. She likely crawled and walked on the wooden floors of her parents' home on Odell Street in Jackson. She may have played with dolls and stuffed animals her parents gave her. Dianne probably babbled sweet baby talk that delighted her doting mother and father. By all accounts, Dianne was a happy, healthy toddler.

In 1950 when Dianne was three years old, she contracted bulbar polio, now called Bulbo-spinal polio. Polio epidemics swept through the United States in the first half of the 20th century. The year Dianne got sick, nearly 34,000 children were paralyzed by polio in the U.S. The poliovirus attacks nerve cells in the brain and spinal cord that control muscle movement, often leading to paralysis. In Dianne's case, the polio damaged the nerves that controlled her breathing muscles. At the time, polio was untreatable. Many children died, while others faced lifetime paralysis and disability.

Within days of noticing Dianne's first symptoms, her frantic parents rushed her to St. Mary's Catholic hospital in Jackson. Doctors placed Dianne in an iron lung, a long metal cylinder that encased her entire body up to her head. The iron lung used alternating pressure to push and pull air in and out of Dianne's paralyzed lungs. The machine enabled her to breathe and saved her life, but she lacked the strength or lung capacity to breathe unassisted. Doctors told her parents that Dianne would likely live only a few weeks at most.

Bringing Dianne Home

After six months at St. Mary's, Freeman and Geneva faced an agonizing decision; bring Dianne home to die or leave her at the hospital indefinitely. The bulky iron lung presented huge logistical hurdles to providing round-the-clock care at home. What's more, no one could predict how long Dianne might linger with her severe breathing challenges. Nevertheless, Freeman and Geneva chose to devote themselves fully to their daughter's care. They felt deep in their souls that Dianne belonged at home.

In early 1951, the Odells arranged the move home for Dianne. The local fire department transported the heavy iron lung to the family's modest house. Every room now centered around 3-year-old Dianne lying motionless in her metal cocoon. The iron lung occupied most of Dianne's bedroom. The Odells set up a mirror above the lung so Dianne could see visitors. Her parents moved Dianne's bed, the iron lung, and its motorized pumps into the living room each day so she could be part of family life.

The Odell house came alive with nurses, physical therapists, and other helpers arriving daily to tend to Dianne's needs. But her parents provided most of her care themselves, feeding her, reading to her, singing with her, praying over her. The Odells remained

steadfast in their commitment to Dianne in defiance
of the grim prognosis.

Precarious Existence

Dianne's survival remained tenuous for many years.
Any electrical outage or equipment failure could be
fatal if the iron lung stopped functioning. Dianne's
father Freeman installed a back-up generator to
power the iron lung in case of electrical failure. The
first big power outage came in 1957, leaving Dianne
dependent on her mother Geneva hand-pumping the
bellows of the iron lung for three hours until
electricity returned.

Another life-threatening power loss happened on
Christmas eve in 1974 during a major winter storm.
Forty-four-year-old Freeman tirelessly hand-pumped
the iron lung again for hours until trucks arrived with
a generator. Other respiratory illnesses and infections
also threatened Dianne's fragile health throughout her

life. Her dependence on the iron lung was absolute; it pumped the air that kept her alive. But Dianne persevered, defying the doctor's early doubts.

Isolation and Changing Times

In the early 1950s, fear of contagion led health officials to discourage polio survivors from public contact. Concerns eased substantially by 1955 when widespread polio vaccination began. However, the ongoing logistics of moving Dianne limited outings. As she grew older, even traveling to another room became impossible without sliding her entire bed base out of the iron lung's narrow opening. Lifting Dianne posed the dangers of equipment disconnections and fractures stemming from childhood polio damage. Despite changing public attitudes, Dianne remained housebound.

As years passed, smaller portable breathing devices replaced bulky iron lungs for most patients. But

Dianne could never switch machines. Severe spinal curvature from polio weakened her back, preventing her from wearing heavy chest devices. While design improved most polio survivors' mobility and independence, Dianne remained reliant on the ever-more-obsolete iron lung technology.

Her unchanged needs amid modernization's march highlighted Dianne's plight. Once numbering in the thousands, only 39 polio survivors in the U.S. still used iron lungs by 1959. By age 15, Dianne was likely one of very few in America who still required 24/7 iron lung support. Yet, her family rose to meet the perpetual challenges of her care.

Family Priorities Shift

As Dianne grew up, life in the Odell home revolved around her illness. Her former bed/playroom overlooked the backyard, filled with children's laughter and play when Dianne was small. But it now

served only Dianne's medical needs, holding IV
stands, suction machines, and other equipment
sustaining the permanent patient within the hulking
iron cylinder.

Dianne's parents forfeited their freedom to give their
daughter as full a home life as possible. They took
turns going to church or stepping out so someone
always remained vigilant at Dianne's side. Financial
hardship from staggering medical bills led them to
plant vegetables rather than flowers. Gone were
thoughts of vacations, dining out, or frivolous
purchases. Each family activity is now factored into
Dianne's elaborate care logistics. Their focus stayed
simply on maintaining 14 Odell Street as Dianne's
sanctuary.

Teenage Dianne

Against all odds, Dianne Odell lived on as a witty, bright teenager. She matured within her family circle, engaging with caregivers and relatives through her angled bedroom mirror. Though the ceaseless whooshing of the ventilation bellows provided her only soundtrack, she grew to young womanhood in her parents' steadfast care.

At 18, Dianne's peers graduated high school and left Jackson for college or jobs. But Dianne could share in none of those rites of passage. Indeed, her entire adolescent social circle disappeared overnight. Still, despite confinement, Dianne began contemplating how to shape her future. Loneliness likely challenged her, with caregivers now comprising her main companions. But demonstrating enormous inner resolve, Dianne started exploring life beyond her four walls.

Seeking Education

Dianne set her sights on finishing high school despite lacking the ability to physically attend classes. Fortunately, times had begun changing. Grassroots disability advocacy now pushed educators towards inclusiveness, not exclusion. So, Dianne asked Jackson Central-Merry High School leaders if she could participate from home. Moved by her plight, they agreed. Teachers shuttled Dianne's assignments and test papers to and from her house. Classmates likely made visits to summarize lessons and lend fellowship. Dianne played exam tapes into a Dictaphone, giving her a voice in school. After years of extraordinary effort, she received her diploma in 1965 at age 18.

Buoyed by this triumph, Dianne soon enrolled in Jackson's Freed-Hardeman University extension courses. College credit seemed impossible for someone who couldn't freely read or write. But

Dianne was undeterred. Freed-Hardeman, inspired by her moxie, delivered course materials and accepted her Dictaphone-submitted work. However, complications from post-polio syndrome soon forced Dianne to halt her studies.

Though she earned no actual degree, Freed-Hardman's president awarded Dianne an honorary bachelor's diploma in 1987 to recognize her remarkable persistence. For Dianne, education's empowerment and self-definition outweighed the diplomas earned. Just grasping each new goal kept her spirit soaring.

Faith Life & The Church of Christ

Dianne grew up in a faithful West Tennessee family active in the Churches of Christ. This Protestant fellowship centers around biblical study, prayer, and hymn singing rather than structured liturgy. Congregants see themselves as part of Christ's universal church but fellowship in local assemblies like Dianne's Jackson church home.

Despite her stillness in the iron lung, Dianne remained vitally engaged in her church community's spiritual life. Sunday services, normally a joyous gathering time for believers, instead came to Dianne through phone lines installed by her father. This innovation allowed the Odells to alternate attending church in person while the other stayed home with Dianne.

The family also actively participated in outreach through the West Jackson Church of Christ. Younger female congregants especially took a shine to nurture the witty iron lung-enclosed woman they called "Sister Dianne." Their regular visits decreased Dianne's sense of isolation and enriched her social connections. Beyond spiritual encouragement, these church friends likely updated Dianne on community happenings. They surely laughed together and forged a touchpoint to a world beyond Dianne's room.

Dianne particularly relished contributing to ministry work by telephoning shut-ins. These faithful ladies and gentlemen, though fully ambulatory, also faced limitations in interacting with their church. Bonding with fellow homebound believers added meaning to Dianne's days despite her greater physical constraints. The church community sustained Dianne's spirit throughout her life.

Dianne's Writing Life

Dianne discovered her latent talent for writing in her 30s. Despite her highly limited mobility, she taught herself to inscribe full sentences letter-by-letter using pens tucked between her toes. Writing this way proved laborious; each special occasion card to friends required hours to compose. But Dianne found the effort worthwhile to connect beyond spoken words. She shared jokes, poetry, encouragement, and holiday greetings via her painstaking script.

This determination to express herself in writing led Dianne to author a children's book decades later. By slowly typing with a mouth stick on voice recognition software, she wrote and self-published "Blinky, Less Light" in 2001. This story shares a tiny star's adventures wishing on a "wishing star" that twinkles less brightly than other stars. Dianne's empathy for difference and disability shines through this allegorical tale about a heroic little star. She dedicated Blinky's story to all children facing challenges.

Book sales provided minimal income to Dianne. But she achieved enormous personal satisfaction revealing creativity hidden inside her iron cage. Despite the great effort required, this unexpected career as an author proved uplifting. Dianne's shining spirit could not be contained even if her body remained motionless.

Recognitions

Word spread in media circles of Dianne's inspirational life. National publications like Woman's World shared her against-the-odds upbringing and achievements. This led to unexpected brushes with celebrity in Dianne's middle age. Actress Jane Seymour highlighted Blinky the wished-upon star while discussing Dianne in her 2004 memoir. Around this time, actor Christopher Reeve also visited Dianne to recognize her courage and perseverance.

Closer to home, Jackson residents celebrated their favorite daughter Dianne's grit despite decades out of public view. Local Rotarians granted her the Paul Harris Fellowship Award, conferred internationally to outstanding humanitarians. Attention grown from her writing won Dianne recognition at holiday events too. Each year at Christmas time, the town welcomed her as a guest of honor at tree-lightings and Nutcracker pageants.

Planning something unique to mark Dianne's 60th birthday in 2007, Jackson leaders decided to hold a grand hotel gala. Transporting Dianne and her massive iron lung to the ballroom required intricate coordination. But townspeople gladly donated furnishings, food, decorations, and entertainment to celebrate Dianne's diamond year. Nearly 200 well-wishers attended the milestone fête with a colossal birthday cake on hand.

These public honors delighted the once-forgotten figure who spent years unseen. Fame seemed irrelevant to quotes attributed to self-effacing Dianne though. She remarked simply that recognition might inspire other disabled individuals. Typically, she focused concern outward, not on herself.

Constant Care Over 60 Years

Behind the scenes, Dianne's family undertook herculean efforts daily to sustain her fragile health over six decades. Freeman installed ceiling tracks above Dianne's iron lung to enable moving her immobilized body for hygiene care. Geneva, retired from teaching to serve as Dianne's primary caregiver, tended to these intimate needs several times a day.

Together the Odells manually retracted the lung's gasket seal and slid Dianne out on a wheeled gurney. Working quickly before Dianne's limited respiratory reserves faltered, they completed arduous cleansing, skin checks, and clothing changes. This routine followed Dianne from infancy to later adulthood, with her parents devoted protectively to preserving her wellness despite the grinding toll of their own advancing age.

Coping With Advancing Age

Time inevitably diminished the Odells' capacities even as Dianne's needs persisted undiminished. Her mother Geneva struggled with arthritis and other aging issues in Dianne's 50s. As her strength to assist Dianne waned, the responsibility shifted to Freeman, himself approaching 80 years old. Severe dementia ultimately forced Geneva's move to assisted living, leaving Freeman as Dianne's sole caregiver.

Meanwhile, Dianne herself experienced post-polio complications increasing her disability. She endured heightened fatigue, joint degeneration, and recurring hospitalizations battling pneumonia. Thankfully a few years prior, the Odells had accepted offers of nursing assistance at home. Rotating private aides spelled Freeman's solo caregiving and kept Dianne from institutionalization. These attendants sustained the Odells' mission to shelter Dianne safely at home no matter what challenges mounted.

For a brief period, the Odell daughters Donna and Mary Beth also assisted their ailing sister. But these working women could not long neglect their own families to replicate their parents' full-time dedication. Dianne's care persisted as a relentless, intimate reality almost impossible for proxy caregivers to maintain. Still, with supplementary medical support and equipment financing through Tennessee's healthcare safety net, father Freeman carried on as Dianne's rock until the night the lights went out for good.

The Night the Lights Went Out

On May 28, 2008, tragedy struck the Odell home. An early summer thunderstorm rumbled through Jackson, downing power lines in Dianne's neighborhood shortly after midnight. Suddenly the motors cycling Dianne's iron lung fell eerily silent. Seconds ticked by agonizingly until emergency lighting activated and the backup generator should have kicked in. But on this fateful night, equipment failure doomed Dianne.

The phone soon jangled urgently at Will Beyer's bedside. Sister Donna Odell Beyer pleaded for Will to rush to Dianne's side at once. A crisis unfolded that demanded every family member's aid. Throwing on clothes, Will raced his pickup through debris-littered streets to the darkened Odell home. Inside, panic reigned. Eighty-two-year-old Freeman labored furiously pumping emergency bellows attempting to oxygenate unconscious Dianne manually. Without powered airflow, mere minutes remained before she would suffocate.

Will desperately fiddled with ignition switches to revive the generator, but it failed to start. Even the antiquated hand crank mechanism could not override the mechanical issues. Helpless, Will too began pumping Dianne's ventilation bag hoping to buy rescuers time. But despite their Herculean efforts, no patchwork actions could sustain Dianne's vital functions any longer. Around 4:00 am with the storm still raging outside, Dianne Odell slipped away peacefully cradled between her father and brother-in-law.

The county sheriff responding later could only confirm Dianne's passing and begin notifying concerned outsiders. For decades, caring for Dianne had defined daily existence for family, friends, and an entire community. Now in the gloomy early hours, the Odells began grieving their beloved girl in the iron lung.

Saying Goodbye

Memorial gatherings filled with tears ensued for beloved Dianne after 62 years in Jackson, Tennessee. The local paper eulogized Dianne poignantly as "a light that shined... an iron will and bottomless well of faith." Townspeople exchanged stories about her unconquerable spirit despite paralysis and isolation. Even in death, Dianne Odell awed others by transcending severe limits on mobility to nurture creativity. She connected intimately with individuals and the community to lead a rich emotional life from surroundings sterile but for family love.

Mourners echoed Dianne's legacy as one who cherished laughter, warmth, and high purpose, not loss over misspent freedoms. People far beyond Jackson wrote the Odells too commiserating over Dianne's profound impact on their lives. Though seldom seen publicly after childhood, in adulthood, her welcoming mirror gaze and breathy speech touched many from her mechanized backdrop.

After her burial, Dianne's bedroom stood vacant for the first time in over half a century, still dominated by the metal ventilator that had encapsulated her world.

In the silence, her family now confronted their profound loss alongside relief from relentless caretaking. Only a lifetime of cherished memories with adventurous, vibrant Dianne could comfort them.

The Odell family's sacrifices to shelter Dianne at home until the end attracted admiration mixed with incredulity. Even as times and technology progressed, they resisted every pressure to institutionalize her. Instead, the Odells reinvented family life around meeting Dianne's needs come what may. They forged partnerships, secured financing, and innovated solutions, but never considered placing her long-term into any hands but their own. This dedication went far beyond medical maintenance to nurture Dianne's emotional health too. Their protectiveness ensured she enjoyed life's pleasures despite missing typical mobility and independence.

As news spread of Dianne's passing, accolades poured in celebrating decades of unwavering love bestowed by her relatives. Freeman and Geneva especially drew praise for eschewing personal freedom to gift their daughter community and togetherness. Local leaders considered the Odell home a monument to family devotion heedless of crushing sacrifice. They praised Dianne's parents for serving as pioneering disability advocates well before the government recognized any supportive infrastructure.

Thanks to the Odell family's extraordinary commitment, Dianne spent over half a century safe at home. She missed no milestone nor any family celebration despite confinement to an iron cylinder since kindergarten. Her parents, rather than yielding to societal indifference about their daughter's welfare, created possibilities unimagined for someone so medically fragile. They painstakingly built physical and emotional access to allow Dianne's participation in wider opportunities. Sadder realities of isolation, loss, anger, and sorrow also accompanied Dianne's journey. But the Odells' priorities kept community and meaning foremost in her existence. They celebrated Dianne's vibrant personhood beyond any disability.

The Ultimate Sacrifice

Inevitably, Dianne's needs finally overtook her elderly father's ability to fulfill them. After Dianne's death, Freeman was likely exhausted from solo caregiving years beyond reasonable capacity. At times he perhaps resented destiny's weight upon his family despite their steadfast Christian faith. The night the power failed; he gave every last ounce to preserve Dianne's precious breath. But his health was doubtless declining too. In the end, their loving daughter Dianne is required to surrender Freeman as well.

Some conjecture the emergency generator's failure resulted from inadequate maintenance. The Odell family could no longer afford proper upkeep of equipment keeping Dianne alive. Did despair or financial realities finally limit their care standards? After so long battling disability day and night, what combination of logistical and emotional burdens finally broke their capacity to preserve Dianne's life above all else? Her death was ruled accidental. But only the Odells know if they had reached their limit playing odds against likely tragedy.

Dianne's Legacy

Thanks to an influx of donated money, Dianne spent nearly all her life in the family home filled with laughter, friendship, and meaning. Her parents' complete commitment to her care there Posts chronicling Dianne's life attracted renewed attention after her passing. Through online dialogue, hundreds of families shared their disability journeys. Dianne's story stimulated conversation about societal duty beyond medical stabilization. It highlighted the support needed so entire families can thrive alongside disability without forfeiting every other priority.

Inspired by the Odells, grassroots disability advocates began calling for expanded school inclusion, accessible housing, and community engagement options. They cited Dianne as evidence that given assets enabling participation, those with even profound disabilities can lead mentally and spiritually whole lives. Dianne proved physical limits need not constrain life's richness.

This activist momentum continues building even 15 years after Dianne's death. Today Dianne Odell remains renowned through books and films documenting her extraordinary story. She endures as the indomitable girl in the iron lung who wrote books, befriended movie stars, and inspired lasting social change; achieving all these without ever taking one step beyond her front door.

Conclusion

As we close the final chapter of " Untold Stories From The Iron Lung: Courageous True Tales of Six Polio Survivors Who Defied the Odds," we are enveloped by a profound sense of awe and reverence for the indomitable human spirit that has permeated the pages of this remarkable journey. From the humble beginnings of the iron lung to its evolution into a symbol of hope and resilience, the stories of courage, perseverance, and triumph have left an indelible mark on our hearts and minds.

Through the archives of history, the iron lung has stood as a silent witness to the triumphs and tribulations of the human experience. It has borne witness to the darkest hours of despair and the brightest moments of hope, serving as a steadfast companion to those grappling with the cruel hand of fate. In the quiet chambers of hospitals and the bustling streets of cities, the iron lung has been a beacon of light in the darkest of times, offering solace and sanctuary to those teetering on the brink of life and death.

As we reflect on the stories of Paul Alexander, Adolf Ratzka, Mona Randolph, Audrey King, Thomas Fetterman, Dianne Odell, and countless others whose lives have been touched by the iron lung, we are reminded of the resilience and strength that lies within each one of us. Their journeys stand as testimonies to the power of the human spirit to overcome adversity, to defy the odds, and to emerge victorious in the face of seemingly insurmountable challenges.

For Paul Alexander, the iron lung has been a faithful companion on a journey fraught with uncertainty and fear. Through the long days and endless nights, he has found solace and comfort within its confines, his unwavering spirit serving as a beacon of hope for all who know his story. In the quiet moments of reflection, he has found strength in the knowledge that he is not alone—that his struggles are shared by countless others who have walked this path before him.

For Mona Randolph, the iron lung has been a silent sentinel against the ravages of disease, standing as a symbol of resilience and determination in the face of adversity. Through the darkest hours of despair, she has found courage and grace within its walls, her unwavering faith guiding her through the storm. In the depths of her struggle, she has discovered a strength she never knew she possessed—a strength forged in the fires of adversity and tempered by the trials of life.

For Philip Drinker and Louis Agassiz Shaw, the iron lung has been a symbol that represents the power of resourcefulness in the face of misfortunes. In the wake of a devastating polio outbreak, they turned to their ingenuity and creativity to craft a viable iron lung that would save countless lives. Through tireless efforts and unwavering determination, they showed us that even in the murkiest of times, there is always hope.

For Dianne Odell, the iron lung was her sanctuary in a world torn apart by diseases and injustice. In the comforting silence of its embrace, she found solace and strength during interminable days and agonizing nights. Her unwavering spirit became a beacon for those touched by her story. Dianne is an embodiment of the unyielding strength and resilience that dwells within us all.

As we bid farewell to the dark era of the iron lung, we are reminded of the enduring power of the human spirit to overcome adversity, to defy the odds, and to emerge victorious in the face of impossible challenges. In the pages of this book, we found solace and sanctuary, strength and resilience, hope and triumph. And though the legacy of the people featured in it may fade over time, their lessons will live on in the hearts and minds of all who have been touched by their remarkable journey.

Ultimately, the measure of our life lies not in its length, but in its richness. As we turn the final pages of this book, let its message linger within our hearts. May we carry forward the lessons etched upon its pages: courage that kindles hope, perseverance that conquers adversity.

Bibliography

1. Kirby, Richard R. (1985). Mechanical Ventilation. New York: Churchill Livingstone. ISBN 978-0443080630.

2. Geddes, LA. (2007). "The history of artificial respiration". IEEE Engineering in Medicine and Biology Magazine, 26(6), 38–41. doi:10.1109/EMB.2007.907081. PMID 18189086. S2CID 24784291.

3. Langmore, Diane (Ed.). (2009). Australian Dictionary of Memoir Volume 17 1981–1990 A–K. Carlton, Victoria: Melbourne University Publishing. ISBN 978-0522853827.

4. Failure in Acute Poliomyelitis". Critical Care and Resuscitation, 8(4), 383–385. PMID 17227281.

5. Silver, Julie K.; Wilson, Daniel J. (2007). Polio Voices. Santa Barbara: Praeger Publishers. p. 141. ISBN 9780275994921.

6. "Artificial Lung on Wheels Prove Life Saver". Popular Mechanics, December 1930.

7. "Iron Lung". National Museum of American History. Retrieved July 1, 2011.

8. Choices, Elspeth (2002). Edinburgh: Mainstream Publishing. pp. 51–52. ISBN 978-1840186116.

9. Healey, John (1998). "The Both Sisters and the 'Iron Lung'". South Australian Medical Heritage Society Inc. Retrieved March 10, 2013.